The Breakfast Book

About the author

Amanda Ursell is a qualified dietician and nutritionist. She is regularly seen on GMTV and has presented *Food File* Channel 4, *Eat Up* Channel 4 and most recently. *The Diet Show* for Living. She has her own column in The Style Section of *The Sunday Times* and *Somerfield* magazine. She writes on a monthly basis for *Men's Health* and *GQ Active* as well as regularly contributing to a wide range of other national newspapers and magazines. Previous books include *The Food File A–Z, The Antioxidant Recipe Book* and *Eat to Beat Indigestion.*

The Breakfast Book

Amanda Ursell

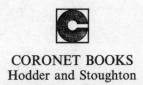

CORONET BOOKS
Hodder and Stoughton

First published in Great Britain in 1998 by Hodder & Stoughton
A division of Hodder Headline PLC

A Coronet Paperback

10 9 8 7 6 5 4 3 2 1

A CIP catalogue record for this title is
available from the British Library

ISBN 0 340 73840 5

Typeset by Hewer Text Ltd, Edinburgh
Printed and bound in Great Britain by
Mackays of Chatham plc, Chatham, Kent

Hodder and Stoughton
A Division of Hodder Headline PLC
338 Euston Road
London NW1 3BH

To my grandparents; for their inspiration,
love and enormous breakfasts

Acknowledgements

There are many people without whom this book would not have been possible. My grateful thanks go to Mark Sims, Eithne Cahill, June Bullock, Jill Niblock, Colin Banks, Rachel O'Connor and Rowena Webb. A huge thanks also to Sarah Such, my editor who so patiently knocked the copy into shape and to Ian Wilson, who has kept the whole project on track and me sane (almost). Also a special thank you to Nick Heath. Finally, a big thanks to all the scientists, past and present, who have helped to prove that breakfast really is the most important meal of the day.

Foreword

I was delighted when Amanda asked me to write a few words about *The Breakfast Book*. Like most of us, the words 'You need a good breakfast inside you' ring in my ears from childhood. Unlike most, I have been privileged to spend a proportion of my working life investigating the science behind the folklore – is there *really* any truth in old adage about the importance of a good breakfast? My answer, as a scientist, is yes my research and that of others has demonstrated time and again that eating the right breakfast improves the diet and so increases your chances of staying healthy and maintaining a healthy body weight.

A good cereal breakfast is, nutritionally, the best possible start to the day – it provides vital vitamins and minerals, and it's low in fat and high in carbohydrate. It can play a significant role in reducing the total fat content of your diet, which is in accordance with current government recommendations. And more than that, the latest research shows that breakfast cereals may actually improve your mental performance. All that in one bowl a day!

The Breakfast Book provides a wealth of information about breakfast, as well as being an entertaining read. I hope it encourages even more of us to make breakfast an essential part of our diet.

Terry Kirk, Senior Lecturer in Nutrition
Queen Margaret College, Edinburgh

Contents

Chapter I

Breakfast like a King

It doesn't matter where in the world you wake up, it's a natural human instinct to want to eat within an hour or two of rising. When you think about it, it's not really that surprising. Having been asleep for probably a good eight hours, and having eaten nothing for perhaps more than ten, your body has undergone a mini fast. Your stomach's completely empty and sending out physical 'I'm hungry' churning sensations. At the same time, your brain knows blood sugar levels are on the lower side of normal and could do with some topping up.

Given these two basic, ancient urges, the physical ones from your stomach and the chemical ones from your brain, it's not surprising those old wives developed a saying to encourage people to tuck into something substantial as their first meal of the day. 'Breakfast like a king, lunch like a knave and dine like a pauper' was how they put it, and it seems that many people are still taking their advice today.

What you eat largely depends on where you live. If it's on the island of Tonga, you might wake up to a substantial *kaipongi-pongi* of ripe bananas, pawpaw and breadfruit. In Honduras your hearty *kesayuno* could be fried kidney beans with eggs, bacon and tortilla, and in the Bahamas your sunrise treat may be something like red snapper and grits.

Going back a bit, say to around 10,000 years BC, man would have eaten anything he could get his hands on and breakfast probably consisted of much the same foods as those eaten during the rest of the day. There wasn't a lot of choice then. Meat from hunting, fish if you were close to rivers or on the sea coasts, and 'vegetables' in the form of wild plants. Women supplemented the diet with anything they could gather, such as snails, small turtles, edible roots, acorns, nuts and berries.

Man's diet changed as he learnt to cook, domesticate animals and grow his own crops. By the time it got to the 1800s, those in Britain who could afford it could expect to be served kidneys, sausages, scrambled eggs and kedgeree at breakfast. For the poor, a chunk of bread or maybe some porridge would be considered a sound start to the day. Across the Atlantic in north America, a gentleman could expect to feast on littleneck clams, mushroom omelettes, grilled plover, and, wait for it, even robins on toast.

As the 1800s moved on, food supplies to towns got better and better, with small farmers supplying milk, cream, butter and eggs and market gardeners bringing in fresh vegetables and fruits. Large-scale production of grains started, and refrigerated rail and sea transport plus improved canning techniques saw the introduction to temperate climates of tropical and subtropical foods. Food companies started to grow and flourish and brand names soon became the rage. Sitting down to something like 'My Lady Fruit Salad' was an incredibly cool thing to do.

The era of food manufacturing had begun, and breakfast in the West was about to undergo a complete revolution as a result. One man was more responsible than anyone else in getting this revolution underway: Will Kellogg.

Chapter 2

The Cereal-makers

Imagine what the typical British breakfast table looked like back in the early 1900s. If well-off, you may have had kedgeree and kippers, piles of bacon, kidneys, fried eggs and bread. Alternatively you could have started your day with some steaming hot porridge. Whatever it was, it was usually hot, as substantial as money allowed, and made by the woman in the house to stoke up her man and her children for the day ahead.

It's perhaps not hard to imagine, therefore, the type of reaction you may have got to the idea of shaking out cereal from a pack, pouring over cold milk and calling it 'breakfast'. My grandma for one was shocked at the prospect. 'The very least I was used to doing was preparing porridge in a double pot over-night,' she said. 'Just putting a suspicious-looking packet of ready-made cereal on the table felt like I was somehow cheating.'

At that time, there were no such things as high-street supermarkets. We were, as Napoleon put it a century before, a nation of shopkeepers. The most you could hope for was a Co-op where you were individually served at separate counters for dairy, meat or bread products, but more likely you bought your supplies in one of the thousands and thousands of tiny traditional corner shops that were often no more than the converted front room of a tiny terraced house overlooking a narrow street.

Changing the breakfast habits of a country used to a daily fry-up in the days when mass marketing was unheard of was one monster task. So just how did it happen? How, in less than a few decades, did we go from saying, 'Corn Flakes – what are they?' to munching our way through millions of packets a year? To find the answer you have to look to the United States, where ready-to-eat cereals were invented. In the latter part of the

1800s, several far-thinking men were working on their own idea of how a cold cereal could be made, what it should be made from and what it should look and taste like.

A Denver lawyer, Henry D. Perky, developed a machine able to press whole grains of wheat into strips, which when baked became the biscuits we know as Shredded Wheat. Perky's invention had been inspired while having lunch at a country inn. As he was deciding what to eat, he noticed a gentleman at a nearby table eating boiled wholewheat mashed with cream – the idea was born. Once he perfected his production techniques, Perky went on to selling his product from a converted wagon in nearby settlements.

While Perky was busy with his wheat cereal, John Stuart, a Scot who emigrated to Canada in 1850, was producing oatmeal for porridge for the local community. Moving to Iowa in the United States, his company formed the Quaker brand of porridge oats, and by the end of the century were also producing puffed wheat and puffed rice which, unlike oats, were designed to be eaten uncooked from the pack: Quaker had already done the cooking for the housewife.

These cereals had in common that their inventors wanted to produce a product that would be healthy to eat. About the same time that these cereals were being introduced to the American public, two brothers, Dr John Harvey Kellogg and Will Harvey Kellogg, were working hard in the Sanatarium in Battle Creek, Michigan. Dr John Harvey Kellogg had taken charge of the Sanatarium, or the 'San', and it was gathering quite a reputation for itself as John Harvey put into practice his new ideas for health reform.

These ideas were based on the theories of Seventh Day Adventists that water treatment, diet, rest, exercise and fresh air were good for people. The ideas seem eminently sensible and acceptable today. Indeed, many people would relish a week of such treatment at health farms like Champney's, Henlow Grange and Greyshott. At the end of the nineteenth century, however, Dr Kellogg was way ahead of his time.

From the word go, he urged his patients to stop smoking, having linked the habit to lung cancer a good half-century before the health risks of smoking became generally accepted. He also persuaded them to count calories. His principles for restoring health were simple and included, among other things, good food. As John Harvey applied his principles of good health to his patients, Will was putting in 120-hour weeks handling the thirty or so extra companies set up by his brother, including everything from publishing to social improvement schemes, from schools and colleges to an orphanage.

The brothers' relationship wasn't always easy but they found time within this frenetic organization to work together in developing new foods for their patients. It was in 1894, while seeking a more digestible substitute for bread, that they accidentally 'invented' another cereal breakfast food.

The Invention of Corn Flakes

The Kellogg brothers had been working on a way to flake wheat by putting boiled grains through heavy rollers. One weekend, while preparing to pass the cooked wheat through the rollers, they were called away on other matters. Left unattended for two days, the wheat almost dried out. The brothers decided to run it through the rollers anyway to see what would happen. What came out was not the long, flat sheets of dough they had expected, but thin flakes. Each wheat kernel had been flattened into a small sliver of grain. Once toasted, these wheat flakes became crisp and light. The first toasted, flaked cereal had been born. Realizing their invention might be popular, they quickly patented the idea and went into limited production.

These original Granose Flakes, as they called them, were not as light and delicate as today's flaked cereals but they represented a breakthrough in cereal technology. The San patients tried them out and, fortunately for the Kellogg brothers, gave them a hearty thumbs-up. So too did former patients, who insisted on buying packets of Granose Flakes mail order from the San. Before long demand outstripped production.

Full of enthusiasm and fired on by the demand, Will and John Harvey started flaking corn, barley and other cereals and began to create a range of health foods for the sanatorium. Between 1895 and 1905 they developed around a hundred health foods. It is the Kelloggs who can be thanked by all peanut butter lovers, for they invented that too!

Before the turn of the century, the first wheat-flaking factory was opened in Battle Creek. Although many others jumped on the bandwagon and tried to copy the Kellogg brothers, few succeeded. Around this time, Will and John Harvey decided to go their separate ways. John Harvey continued his work at the San, while Will started the Toasted Corn Flake Company (later to become Kellogg's). It was at this time that Will Kellogg turned his back on flaked wheat, choosing instead to concentrate on flaking corn. He was soon shown to have backed the winner although at the time, to a sceptical American nation, corn meant horse food.

Herein lay one of the main differences between Will Kellogg and his competitors. Will Kellogg had a flaked cereal and it was made not from wheat or oats but corn. Experiments to get his corn flakes just right involved the use of corn grits instead of whole corn and the addition of malt and sugar. After all, we were all adding sugar and salt to porridge, so why shouldn't corn get a helping hand?

The other main difference was his extraordinary drive and determination, something only the most successful entrepreneurs have. Will Kellogg took his health food and turned it into an everyday breakfast, convincing the American nation that this was the way they should start their day.

Changing a Nation's Breakfast Habits

Will Kellogg set out on a mission to improve the health of the American nation. His career had had an unlikely start. At the tender age of fourteen he worked in his father's company selling brooms. At the age of twenty he left the brooms behind him, married his childhood sweetheart and took himself off to business school. This background in sales and business was to prove invaluable.

Against all the rules, Will Kellogg invested heavily in advertising and promoting Corn Flakes. In addition to a huge advertising push, he launched a city-wide sampling programme which was, quite literally, done door to door. With these two techniques he set in motion the cereal revolution in the United States. Will Kellogg did for breakfast cereals what Henry Ford did for cars. He marketed them brilliantly and grew the marketplace for everyone.

His techniques worked. Demand went completely bananas. In 1907 he famously uttered the words, 'Now we can turn out forty-two hundred cases a day and that's all the business I ever want.' By 1920 output had increased to 24,000 cases a day.

The Atlantic Crossing

The first taste the British got of these strange, new, ready-to-eat cereal foods was after the turn of the twentieth century. Quaker's Puffed Wheat and Puffed Rice made their way to our shores in 1907 and 1910 respectively. In 1908, Shredded Wheat appeared in London. The first time we got a sniff of Corn Flakes was when American soldiers joined the war effort in Europe towards the end of the First World War and brought packets with them, which a favoured few got to sample.

With a sincere belief in the quality and value of their product, Kellogg's officially brought Corn Flakes to Britain in 1922. The Kellogg's company hit our shores running, applying the same marketing principles they had so successfully started in the States a few decades before. Within months they had hired a top-rate sales team who would do the same corner-shop-to-corner-shop legwork that had so dramatically changed America's breakfast table.

Getting on with the Legwork

Archie Mountford, one of the highly motivated team of salesmen who put Corn Flakes and the new product All-Bran on our nation's morning menu, had his work cut out. 'In my early days

I worked on foot. Each salesman was provided with a large hide case, very heavy even when empty, which contained samples, collapsed dummy packets for display, price tickets, crepe paper, drawing pins, order book, credit book, report book and other sundry documents. In addition we were sent large quantities of cardboard cut-outs for display purposes, and these had to be made up into brown-paper parcels and carried each day.

'And so I set off – just a typical day – loaded down with my luggage but hopeful that early on I would find a grocer who would allow me to clear part or the whole of a window or convenient display point in order to promote sales – and also to lighten my load.

'To preserve some semblance of respectability, before entering a shop I used to leave the brown-paper parcel outside, if possible behind a placard in case of rain or the attention of passing dogs. On this day it had rained so the parcel was already a mess when I called at a shop in the early afternoon. This shop had no outside protection for my parcel so I just had to take a chance. By now quite demoralized but still determined, I tried the hard sell again. No hope. I left the shop with my tail between my legs. I was very near the River Thames by now and I debated whether to throw myself, the parcel, or both into the river. I finally discovered a small shop whose proprietor listened to my pleas and he got tremendous window display!'

Sometimes things got really tough. Another retired salesman recalls: 'More cereals meant less bacon, and one very irate grocer waved a nasty-looking bacon-slicing knife under my nose and told me to stop talking about these blankety-blank Corn Flakes and get out of his blankety-blank shop before he sliced me up for his blankety-blank customers.'

As salesmen tramped the streets with their products, talking their way past the counters and on to the shelves and display areas of countless thousands of shops, the same door-to-door sampling that Kellogg's carried out in the United States took place in our streets. Kellogg's men became welcome faces at Labour Exchanges, where casual workers were hired for six shillings a day to fill their bags with eighty sample packets at a time and hand them out with leaflets to housewives. With a horse and cart pulling the reserve sample packs, teams of workers (and sometimes Boy Scouts) were putting Corn Flakes into the hands of often suspicious users for the very first time.

Between 1925 and 1931 sales in Britain rose fivefold and in the 1930s they increased tenfold. In 1936 some one million cases of Corn Flakes had been sold in the UK. Four hundred thousand packets a week were at this stage being shipped over from Canada. Head office in Battle Creek realized Britain needed its own manufacturing plant and so it came to pass.

Making our Own

The plant was built in Stretford, Manchester. In April 1938 the first pack of Corn Flakes rolled off the production line. Employees could expect to take home good wages of one to three shillings per hour. By 1939, the workforce had increased to some 250 and it was time for the official opening. The managing director, Harry McEvoy, and his colleagues dreamt up the idea of having a typical British housewife to do the honours.

The search was on. Out of 5,000 entrants, Mrs Florence May Millward, a 45-year-old miner's wife from Mansfield, was chosen. Somehow she managed to bring up six children aged four to twenty on her husband's wage of under three pounds a week. In her opening speech she declared that, in her opinion, the consuming of cereals was necessary for the health of the people. Pretty much what Will and John Harvey had felt and subsequently promoted some forty years earlier at the Battle Creek San. She felt sure that all who knew the merits of the Kellogg's products would continue to purchase them regularly.

She wasn't wrong. Although during the Second World War corn grits ran out and production switched to Wheat Flakes, Kellogg's kept feeding the nation's soldiers with both these and All-Bran. As the War Office cartoons show, they gave their approval for cereals to be included in the regular Army diet.

During the war, when nationwide transport became almost impossible, the cereal manufacturers were allocated parts of the country to supply. Shredded Wheat were awarded London and the south-east, Weetabix the Midlands and Kellogg's the north. And Kellogg's kept telling us what all good housewives knew. You can't do a good day's work without a substantial breakfast.

By the time the war was over, it was no longer a newfangled notion to pour your breakfast cold from a pack. Ready-to-eat breakfast cereals were an established part of the nation's diet and everyone was clamouring for them. When the first corn arrived from Romania a year after the war had ended it was full of army buttons, a sad reminder of the battles that had been fought on the cornfields. By 1947, Corn Flakes were back on the breakfast tables of Britain. Rice took longer to arrive and it was not until May 1951 that Rice Krispies re-appeared, with 21-foot bus posters telling everyone they were back.

Supermarkets and Promotions

In 1951, Britain's first supermarket, the Premier, opened in Streatham Hill, London. Self-service became the rage and the Co-op soon caught on to the new phenomenon.

With the growth in popularity of supermarkets came more sophisticated promotion of breakfast cereals. Kellogg's packets and adverts still carried health messages and remained true to the original Kellogg brothers' philosophy of giving people affordable, nutritious, simple foods.

Notwithstanding this ideal, cereals had to move with the times and soon they were to carry offers of give-away gifts and packet-back cut-outs to entertain children. Who doesn't remember the rush to find the free gift buried deep inside a new box of cereal? Original packet inserts from days gone by are now eagerly sought by collectors.

One Corn Flakes offer in 1957 captured many people's imagination. It was a plastic model of an 'Atomic' submarine. Fuelled by baking powder, it dived and surfaced in a bathful of water much to the fascination of kids, dads, and, it would seem, the Royal Navy itself.

On-pack promotions continue to get huge, and sometimes unexpected, responses.

'Dear Sir,' wrote a fed-up father from Yeovil, 'whilst enjoying my Rice Krispies for breakfast this morning I could not help but notice the offer boldly emblazoned on the packet – 'Jeans for Kids'. I therefore write to you with haste to take advantage of this philanthropic gesture and to inquire how many pairs of jeans you will allow me in exchange for my children, a girl aged 13 and a boy aged 9. Perhaps you would also let me know the means by which I should despatch my children to you, and whether, as some sort of proof of transfer of ownership, you require me to let you have their birth certificates . . .'

Competition

As the biggest cereal producers in the business, Kellogg's expanded the marketplace, which helped other cereal manufacturers to promote their products. Shredded Wheat continued to do well, as did Quaker's products and Weetabix. As market leaders, Kellogg's developed new cereals designed to keep up with demand and satisfy people's different needs. Will Kellogg had set the scene, the public had accepted a cold cereal start to the day, and now they wanted variety. All-Bran had reached us in 1938, Rice Krispies in 1940 and Bran Flakes in 1952.

Competition today is fierce in the breakfast-cereal industry. The ready-to-eat cereal market in Britain is now worth approximately £950 million a year. Kellogg's have almost 40 per cent of the market, 'others' – meaning own brands – 31 per cent, Weetabix 14 per cent, Cereal Partners UK (Shredded Wheat, Shredded Wheat Fruitful, Honey Shredded Wheat, Clusters, Golden Grahams, Fibre 1 and Cheerios) 12 per cent, and Quaker almost 3 per cent.

According to 1996 figures, these were the most popular brands in the UK.

Britain's Most Popular Brands

Cereal	£ sales 1996	Company
1. Kellogg's Corn Flakes	Over 99 million	Kellogg
2. Weetabix	70–75 million	Weetabix
3. Kellogg's Frosties	60–65 million	Kellogg
4. Kellogg's Rice Krispies	35–40 million	Kellogg
5. Kellogg's Crunchy Nut Corn Flakes	35–40 million	Kellogg
6. Kellogg's Bran Flakes	30–40 million	Kellogg
7. Nestlé Shredded Wheat	25–30 million	Cereal Partners
8. Kellogg's Coco Pops	25–30 million	Kellogg
9. Kellogg's Special K	25–30 million	Kellogg
10. Kellogg's Fruit 'n Fibre	25–30 million	Kellogg

Today there is a breakfast cereal brand for everyone. From Crunchy Nut Corn Flakes to Alpen, from Sustain to Weetabix.

How Cereals help get Messages across

Despite its commercial success and long before healthy eating became popular, Kellogg's stuck to its founders' guiding beliefs in the importance of a balanced diet and busily went about letting the public know of current health thinking. As early as the 1940s they devised games for teachers to use when explaining nutrition to younger children. In the 1950s newspaper advertisements illustrated educational features and explained the dietary value of breakfast, and in a 1970s television commercial Kellogg's emphasized the vitamins and iron in Corn Flakes through a song, 'It's smart to start your day the Kellogg's Corn Flakes way.'

Today cereal manufacturers are responsible for providing award-winning educational materials in the form of computer programs, health and fitness videos and, last but not least, invaluable on-pack information, read and inwardly digested by millions and millions of people as their packets of cereal sit in front of them at breakfast each morning.

Not only do we read the information but it appears we trust

it. A survey conducted by the Henley Centre, a research and marketing group, suggested that we trust our Corn Flakes more than our MPs. Kellogg's Corn Flakes topped the list of individual products with 84 per cent of the 2,000 sample expressing faith in the brand and thus its on-pack messages. In fact, they believed them more than information supplied by the government, the press and even the church.

This trust in Kellogg's messages is great news for the organizations with whom cereal manufacturers choose to work to get health messages across. Organizations such as Breakthrough Breast Cancer, who have produced a joint leaflet with Kellogg's to raise awareness of breast cancer detection and prevention. During National Breakfast Week, the partnership managed to raise nearly £100,000 to boost the charity's funds. Good news too for the Cancer Research Campaign, who have had their bowel-cancer prevention messages put on over a million packs of All-Bran as part of a nationwide campaign to increase awareness.

When the Health Education Authority decided to launch a folic acid campaign and to use cereals to promote their 'With Extra Folic Acid' label, millions of women of childbearing age got the message – that taking extra folic acid in fortified cereals and supplement form before becoming pregnant can greatly reduce the risk of having a baby with spina bifida (see Chapter 7).

A good century after their development, ready-to-eat breakfast cereals are not only still with us but are playing a vital role in our diet. Those health-reforming cereal entrepreneurs of the late 1800s, would be proud to see that their cereal revolution is continuing, quite literally, to improve the health of nations.

Chapter 3

Nutrition – Getting the Facts Straight

'Breakfast consumption, particularly if the meal includes a breakfast cereal, is associated with lower intakes of fat and higher intakes of carbohydrate, dietary fibre and certain micronutrients.' So says a scientist writing in the *British Journal of Nutrition*.

It seems like the author of this piece is backing breakfast, but just what exactly does all that business of fat, carbohydrate, fibre and 'certain micronutrients' actually mean? We have words like these thrown at us every day: in newspapers, magazines on television, and on the nutrition labels crammed on to every packet of food and drink in the supermarket.

Here's a crash course so you can bone up on the basics of nutrition.

Why Do We Need to Eat and Drink?

Just like animals, we need to eat and drink to live – to grow, to maintain our bodies once we are fully grown and to reproduce. With the advances of modern nutritional science it has become clear that the kind and quantity of foods and drink we consume affects us from the moment of conception through to old age.

If the food and drink we put into our bodies is not enough or of poor quality, we start to suffer. It may be simply that we don't reach our maximum potential height because we didn't get enough food as youngsters. It may be that we develop weak bones in later life because we didn't eat enough of the right things as a teenager. On the other hand, perhaps we've ended up eating too much, causing overweight and leading to problems with joints, varicose veins and the heart – not to mention how we feel about ourselves.

Eating the right amount and the right quality of food allows us to maximize what we've inherited in our genes from our parents. The food we eat is eventually reflected in the health of our bones, muscle, skin, hair, teeth, brain and every other part of the body you can think of. What we eat can help make us fit and possibly even fight off killer diseases like cancer and heart disease.

So Much Choice – What Should We Eat?

For sheep and cows it's easy. When they are out in the fields there's one choice: grass. They amble around eating all day and, fortunately for them, this satisfies all their nutritional requirements. Lions need to manage a regular kill, and penguins need to catch fresh fish. For man living in the modern Western world, however, it's a different story. Surrounded as we are by thousands and thousands of food products, we need to eat a good balance of what's on offer. Too much and sometimes too little of certain foods can lead to health problems. With all the choices it's easy to get things wrong. Usually not wrong enough to make us look ill from the outside, but often wrong enough for us not to be firing on all cylinders on the inside.

You may find it surprising that the millions of food products on offer in the supermarkets are all made up from just a handful of major nutrients. These are proteins, carbohydrates and fats. Many foods are a mixture of two or more of these plus water, and most foods are also a source of the minor though no less vital nutrients known as vitamins and minerals.

Protein

When the bulk of the food in question supplies protein it's known as a protein-rich food. The ones we're all familiar with are red meat, chicken, turkey, duck, fish, eggs, milk and dairy products. From the vegetable world, soya products, Quorn, nuts and seeds also provide protein.

Every cell in the body needs protein – or rather the amino acids from which protein is made – to keep its structure intact. Yet we need surprisingly little each day: an adult man needs around 55 grams and a woman around 45 grams. There's no point eating lots more since the excess gets broken down and turned into extra calories. (A gram of protein provides 4 calories.) Eating very high-protein diets can actually put a strain on the organs that carry out this breakdown process, and anyway protein foods tend to be the expensive ones, so what's the point in wasting money by eating too much of them?

Food	Serving size	Protein content
Bacon, back	3 rashers	11 grams
Beef	85 grams	24 grams
Chicken breast	85 grams	23 grams
Chicken leg	190 grams (1 leg)	29 grams
Cod	130 grams	27 grams
Duck	85 grams	22 grams
Eggs	2 medium	8 grams
Ham	55 grams (2 slices)	10 grams
Lamb	85 grams	25 grams
Mackerel	110 grams	24 grams
Milk	195 ml (1/3 pint)	6 grams
Milk	115 ml (cereal-bowl size)	4 grams
Peanuts	30 grams (32 nuts)	7 grams
Plaice	120 grams	19 grams
Pork	85 grams	26 grams
Salmon	135 grams	22 grams
Soy beans	100 grams	14 grams
Tofu	100 grams	8 grams
Turkey	85 grams	24 grams
Yoghurt	150 grams	6 grams

Carbohydrates

Carbohydrates include foods such as breakfast cereals, bread, pasta, rice, potatoes, noodles, chapati, couscous, pitta, sweet potato, yams, cassava and plantain (green banana). Along with these are, for example, fruit buns, scones, malt loaf and scotch pancakes. We think of these foods as being 'starchy'. Sugary foods, such as table sugar, honey, sweets like wine gums, fruit pastilles and boiled sweets, and sugary puddings such as meringues are also carbohydrates, as are fruits and vegetables.

Once we have eaten any of these foods, they get broken down into glucose. Glucose is carried around in the blood and used as the energy currency of all cells. This energy powers all the activities that go on inside us minute by minute, hour by hour and day by day. The carbohydrate we don't need gets stored in the muscles and the liver. If we eat way too much carbohydrate, some of the excess gets converted into fat.

Carbohydrate foods supply the body with the same amount of calories per gram as protein. This means that for every gram of carbohydrate you eat you are getting 4 calories. This is true whether the food is starchy or sugary. Starchy carbohydrate foods usually supply the body with quite a lot of vitamins and minerals as well as energy. On average men need to eat about 300 grams of carbohydrates a day, whereas women need about 250 grams.

Food	Serving size	Carbohydrate content
Apple	1	11 grams
Apricots, dried	25 grams (about 3)	11 grams
Banana	1	15 grams
Bread, medium sliced	2 slices	37 grams
Bread, pitta	1	38 grams
Bread roll	55 grams	28 grams
Cereal, bowl of	40 grams	30–40 grams
Coke	330ml	21 grams
Crumpets	2	26 grams
Currant bun	50 grams	26 grams
Fruit pastilles	1 tube	24 grams
Honey	1 teaspoon	5 grams
Malt loaf	2 slices	34 grams
Orange	1	16 grams
Pasta, boiled	150 grams	35 grams
Rice, boiled	165 grams	53 grams
Rye crispbreads	3	17 grams
Scone	1	24 grams
Sugar	1 teaspoon	5 grams
Wine gums	1 tube	13 grams

Fats

This is the third major nutrient group, and has had a lot of bad press over recent years. Just ten years ago the words 'Additive Free' on a pack of food made us want to buy it. These days 'Fat Free' stimulates the same response. Are we getting paranoid about fat?

We probably are, although this paranoia about the word doesn't mean that we're doing anything positive about the problem. In fact, since the Second World War, as a country we have been eating more and more.

So where do we find fats? The most obvious places are in those foods that look and feel fatty. For example, margarine, butter and oil, and fat on meat. However, foods which supply large amounts of fats are not always easy to pinpoint. Take a sausage. Since the sausage meat is wrapped up in a skin, it's impossible to tell that a couple of sausages have the equivalent fat of two tablespoons of butter or margarine.

How about a chicken breast? How are you to know that 12 grams of fat lurk in the skin? Or what about a packet (100 grams) of Bombay mix? That contains 32 grams of fat; a serving of taramasalata contains 46 grams, a small chunk of Cheddar 15 grams and 5 slices of salami 25 grams. It's just that you can't see these large quantities of fat. That's why checking food labels is a good habit to get into.

The big difference between fat, protein and carbohydrate is that, gram for gram, fats supply us with twice the calories. This means that 1 gram of fat supplies the body with 9 calories as opposed to 4. By eating fat-laden foods you get twice the calories you would from protein and carbohydrate foods, so it's much easier to overeat and put on weight. It's recommended that men stick to 90 grams of fat per day and women to 70 grams. If you are trying to lose weight then you can virtually halve these figures. Breakfast can be a virtually fat-free meal or it can be laden with fat. It depends what you choose. Take a look at these figures.

Food	Serving size	Fat content
Corn Flakes with semi-skimmed milk and chopped banana	1 bowl	2 grams
Crisps and chocolate	1 packet and 1 average bar	20 grams
Croissant	2 with butter	40 grams
Danish pastry	1	18 grams
Fry-up	1 fried egg, 3 rashers bacon and 2 slices fried bread	55 grams
Scrambled egg on toast	2 eggs on 2 slices	47 grams
Toast with butter or margarine	2 slices with 20 grams of spread	16 grams

Polyunwhatsits

The problems with fat don't end with its poor rating on the calorie stakes. Not only do we need to cut back on the total amount we eat, we also need to think about the type we eat. This means thinking about where the fat comes from. Is it from an animal source, like the fat in and around a pork chop or the fat in a steak and kidney pie, the skin on your roast chicken or the butter you've slapped on your toast? Or is it instead from the oils found in fish such as tuna and mackerel, and in some nuts, seeds and vegetables? Although weight for weight all fats supply the same calories, your body deals with them differently.

The animal sources are high in what we call saturated fats. These seem to be able to raise cholesterol levels in the blood, which can increase the risk of fatty lumps building up on artery walls. This can make you more prone to heart disease.

Fats from the plant world, on the other hand, tend to be unsaturated and don't have this effect on cholesterol levels in the blood. They also have the advantage of supplying us with so-called 'essential fats', which are vital for the instigation and regulation of many activities in the body. Mums need plenty when pregnant to feed their baby's growing brain; infants need lots to continue this brain growth; kids need them for proper development of sight and hearing, and adults need them for good skin and for hormonal balance.

When you translate all this into daily eating habits, it means you do need some fats every day. Just try to make sure that you stick within the suggested number of grams for your sex, that you cut back on the animal ones to help your heart, and that you include fats from plants and fish so that you're getting the vital 'essential' fats.

Vitamins and Minerals

That's the main nutrients covered, the ones that make up the main bulk of our food. Now it's the turn of the small nutrients, the vitamins and minerals. They are impossible to see but we know they're there. They started to be discovered and pinpointed in the 1700s. You may have heard of the sailors who after months at sea started to suffer from scurvy. Old wounds re-opened, gums bled, teeth fell out and new wounds didn't heal. Eventually internal organs would break down and death could follow. What was the cause of such a nasty condition? Some dreaded tropical disease? No, nothing as exotic as that. It was simply a complete lack of fresh foods in the diet, and therefore an absence of vitamin C. They had no oranges, grapefruit, fresh berries or dark green vegetables to eat. In 1747 a scientist called Lind carried out a test on the sailors on HMS *Salisbury* and discovered that oranges and lemons (good suppliers of vitamin C) prevented scurvy.

Other vitamins and minerals have roles to play in the body just as important at this, and a lack of any of them can lead to a corresponding problem with health. Take a look at the table below.

Vitamins

Vitamin	Where you find it	What it's for	Deficiency
C	Citrus fruits and juices, berries, kiwi fruits, dark green vegetables, peppers	Helps absorb iron from food; maintains healthy skin and gums; an antioxidant	Scurvy
B1	Fortified breakfast cereals, milk, bread, potatoes	Necessary for the release of energy from carbohydrates	Beri-beri (shortage of breath and paralysis)
B2	Fortified breakfast cereals, milk, meat, eggs, vegetables	Important for healthy skin, eyes and nails; helps release energy to cells	Rash around nose and inflammation of the tongue
B6	Fortified breakfast cereals, milk, meat, potatoes and other vegetables	For healthy blood, skin and nerves and proper use of proteins	Inflammation of the tongue, lesions of the lips and nerve damage
B12	Fortified breakfast cereals, milk, cheese, fish, eggs, meat	Helps blood cells grow and develop; important for a healthy nervous system	Pernicious anaemia and nerve damage

Vitamins—*contd*

Vitamin	Where you find it	What it's for	Deficiency
Niacin	Fortified breakfast cereals, milk, cheese, yoghurt, potatoes, bread	Involved in energy-producing reactions in cells	Pellagra, a disease which gives a red rash on the skin, plus diarrhoea and dementia
Folate	Green vegetables, wholemeal bread, Marmite	Essential for growing cells and healthy blood; also important for healthy babies and a healthy heart	Increased risk of having a child with spina bifida; possible increased risk of heart disease; megaloblastic anaemia
Folic acid	Fortified breakfast cereals, fortified bread	As above for folate	As above for folate
D	Fortified breakfast cereals, eggs, butter, fortified margarine, oily fish	Helps the body absorb calcium; needed for strong bones and teeth	Rickets, osteomalacia, osteoporosis, stunted growth
E	Fortified breakfast cereals, seeds, wholemeal cereals, eggs, dark green vegetables, avocados, nuts	To protect cell walls from damage	Nerve damage; possible increased risk of heart disease
A	Liver, whole milk, butter, eggs, fortified margarine, dark green vegetables and carrots, Kellogg's Sustain	Good night sight; keeps membranes moist	Xerophthalmia (a serious eye disorder)

Minerals

Mineral	Where you find it	What it's for	Deficiency
Calcium	Milk, cheese, yoghurt, green vegetables, canned fish with bones, sesame seeds, tahini, All-Bran Plus (fortified with calcium)	Strong bones and teeth; muscle contraction and blood clotting	Rickets, osteoporosis
Iron	Red meat, fortified breakfast cereals, eggs, wholemeal bread, dark green vegetables	Red blood cell formation; health of red blood cells	Anaemia: tiredness, no concentration
Zinc	Shellfish, red meat, Kellogg's Sustain, milk, wholegrain bread	Healthy immune system; good sense of taste; growth; healthy sperm	Impotence, skin problems
Magnesium	Milk, bread, cereals, potatoes, other vegetables	Good muscle tone	Poor nervous system and bones
Potassium	Vegetables and fruit	Control of body water	Weak muscles, confusion
Copper	Wholegrain cereals, meat, vegetables	Immune system and proper growth	Weak bones, susceptibility to infections
Fluoride	Tea, fish, water	Increases resistance to tooth decay	Increased risk of tooth decay

It's uncommon for people in the West to suffer with the extreme deficiency diseases listed here, which are caused by a seriously low intake of vitamins and minerals in their diet. However, it is possible that lowish intakes mean we don't function as optimally as we might. Keeping up our daily intakes is therefore important.

Water

A staggering four-fifths of our bodies is made up of water, which constantly needs to be topped up. We use water on a daily basis for controlling metabolic processes and for keeping ourselves at the correct temperature. We lose it not only through sweating and urination but also in our faeces and through breathing. Depending on how hot and dry it is and how much exercise we do, we need at least one and half litres a day, with another litre for every hour of exercise.

Most of us drink about two litres of fluid a day and take another litre in the food we eat. In hot weather we drink more. It is important to drink plenty. You can tell when you are not drinking enough because your urine is dark-coloured, smells a bit and you don't produce very much of it. When you are drinking enough, your urine will be pale in colour and you'll go to the loo more often. Once you get even slightly dehydrated your body will function less well, so it's vital you keep up your fluids all day. The elderly and young are particularly at risk from not drinking enough.

Fibre

This is the part of plant foods that is not absorbed in the small intestine. If you look at the picture of the digestive system on page 75, you will see the intestine is divided into two parts. The top part is the small intestine, and the bottom part the large intestine or colon. The fibrous part of plant foods doesn't get broken down like protein, fat and carbohydrate in the small intestine but goes on into the large intestine, where it is fermented by the millions of friendly bacteria that live there. The fermentation process bulks out the stools – making them bigger – which gives the colon a good physical workout.

By speeding up the rate at which stools pass through the colon you reduce the risk of constipation. You may also be helping to push through potential cancer-causing substances so they have less chance of setting up cancerous lesions in the colon wall.

Fibre is present in wholewheat products such as wholegrain breakfast cereals like the famous All-Bran, as well as in wholemeal bread, wholewheat pasta, brown rice and pitta bread and brown muffins. Some fruit and vegetables also supply the bulking type of fibre while others, like apples and pears, contain a type of fibre that helps to keep blood cholesterol and sugar levels even. We need to aim for around 18 grams of fibre a day. The best way to achieve this is to eat plenty of wholegrain cereals of all types and to aim to have five servings of fruits and vegetables a day.

Fruits and Vegetables

Although fruits and vegetables have been touched on above under carbohydrates, vitamins and minerals and fibre, they deserve a special mention since, in addition to supplying us with all of these nutrients, they also contain lots of other substances that are thought to help prevent many kinds of diseases. For example, the wonderful red colouring of tomatoes is given by a pigment called lycopene which is thought to play a role in reducing the risk of heart disease. The bright orange beta-carotene pigment so richly found in carrots may help fight lung cancer. And many, many other compounds found in all sorts of fruits and vegetables could play important roles in maintaining the health of everything from our eyes to our skin.

The key is to get a good variety and to try to eat five servings a day. Breakfast is a great place to start, either with a vegetable or fruit juice or with chopped or grated fruit on your cereal (each of which counts as one serving). Alternatively, make up a fresh or winter fruit salad or include some fruit in a whizzed-up milk and yoghurt smoothie.

Summing it all up

A healthy diet is all about getting the balance right. Having enough, not too much or too little, of any particular food or drink means getting the right balance of nutrients. The healthy-eating pyramid provides us with a good visual guide as to how we can achieve this when planning our daily meals and snacks.

The Food Pyramid Guide
A Guide to Daily Food Choices

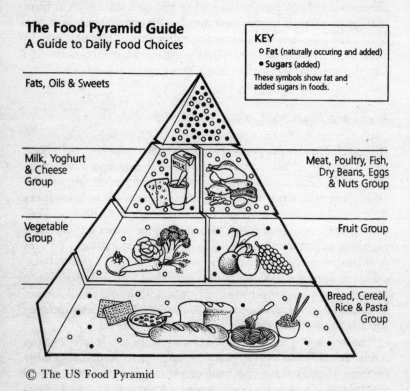

KEY
○ Fat (naturally occuring and added)
● Sugars (added)
These symbols show fat and added sugars in foods.

Fats, Oils & Sweets

Milk, Yoghurt & Cheese Group

Meat, Poultry, Fish, Dry Beans, Eggs & Nuts Group

Vegetable Group

Fruit Group

Bread, Cereal, Rice & Pasta Group

© The US Food Pyramid

Chapter 4

Why a Cereal Start?

There are lots of good reasons for pouring out a bowl of cereal each morning. The chances are you love the taste and have your special favourites. But there are also four really great health reasons, which just goes to show, it doesn't have to be hell to be healthy – sometimes it's actually delicious.

It's Low in Fat

You need to check your favourite pack, but most cereals are very low in fat. If you serve them with skimmed or semi-skimmed milk you can easily have a breakfast with under 5 grams of fat. Experts agree that eating a breakfast which includes a breakfast cereal is associated with lower intakes of fat – and that makes a contribution to *being* less fat.

One pretty good reason for a cereal start.

It's High in Carbohydrates

And here's another. Cereals supply us with both starchy and sugary carbohydrates. These give the body energy to last throughout the morning and supply glucose to the brain to keep us thinking straight. Diets rich in carbohydrates help us to control our body weight and supply us with lots of energy to fuel exercise and play.

It's Rich in Vitamins and Minerals

Besides being low in fat and high in carbohydrate, if you choose carefully a cereal will add significant amounts of vitamins and minerals to your daily intake as well. If you choose cereals fortified with added vitamins and minerals, with just one bowl you can often get at least a third of an adult's and a quarter of a child's requirements of these vital nutrients.

Vitamin D: Helps your body absorb the calcium in milk
Vitamin E: An antioxidant needed to maintain a healthy body and protect cells from damage
Vitamin C: Helps the body absorb iron to keep the blood strong
Vitamins B1, B2: Help convert energy from carbohydrate into a form the body can use
Vitamin B6: Needed for healthy blood and nerves
Vitamin B12: Helps blood cells grow and develop, and is important for a healthy nervous system
Folic acid: Helps keep the blood healthy. You need the greatest amount when trying for a baby because it helps the development of a baby's spinal cord: an extra 400 micrograms a day. Look for cereals with 'Extra Folic Acid'. These supply around 100 micrograms extra per day
Iron: Needed for strong blood
Zinc: Important for a healthy immune system

It Supplies Fibre

Depending on the cereal you choose, you can get anything up to half your day's recommended intake of fibre in just one bowl. The highest in fibre are the cereals made from the whole grain, which means they contain the rough, outside part of the wheat or oat grain. Even the less obviously fibrous cereals still supply the body with important carbohydrate which gets into the colon, is fermented by bacteria and bulks the weight of the stool. The following table shows you the top fibre-providers, and the runners-up.

Cereal	Fibre per 40-gram bowl
All-Bran Plus	12 grams
Fibre 1	12 grams
All-Bran Buds	11 grams
Weetabix Crunchy Bran	11 grams
All-Bran Bite Size	10 grams
Bran Buds	10 grams
Bran Flakes	6 grams
Oat Bran Flakes	5 grams
Sultana Bran	5 grams
Force	4 grams
Frosted Wheats	4 grams
Fruit 'n' Fibre	4 grams
Raisin Wheats	4 grams
Shredded Wheat	4 grams
Weetabix	4 grams
Alpen	3 grams
Country Store	3 grams
Frutibix	3 grams
Multi-Grain Start	3 grams
Shreddies	3 grams
Strike	3 grams
Sustain	3 grams
Muesli	2 grams
Puffed Wheat	2 grams

Comparing Breakfasts

Breakfast	Calories	Fat	Carbo-hydrate	Protein	Fibre
Fruit 'n' Fibre with semi-skimmed milk and chopped banana	303	5 grams	60 grams	9 grams	4 grams
Corn Flakes with grated apple and semi-skimmed milk	273	4 grams	56 grams	8 grams	2 grams
Fried egg, 2 rashers of bacon and fried bread	541	42 grams	19 grams	24 grams	1 gram
Scrambled eggs on 2 slices of toast	603	44 grams	35 grams	19 grams	1 gram
2 slices of toast with butter and honey	364	17 grams	50 grams	6 grams	1 gram

Chapter 5

From Classroom to Boardroom, Breakfast boosts Performance

If at a parents' evening your child's teacher suggested little Johnny's lessons would improve if he paid more attention, you might think, 'I've heard that before.' You'd probably be surprised, however, if the teacher went on to ask if he had a good breakfast before leaving home. You might well feel like responding, 'What's that got to do with you?'

It would have a lot to do with the teacher, since experiments carried out on children both in laboratories and in their own schools indicate that those who skip breakfast or who eat very little at the start of the day are at a disadvantage compared to those who have something 'proper' to eat before leaving home.

How can Breakfast help Performance in School?

It seems to be down to the simple fact that if you have not eaten anything since the night before, by the time morning comes the levels of blood sugar reaching the brain are below optimal. This doesn't mean your kids are going to keel over or fall asleep at their desks. What it could mean, however, is that during the morning's lessons, certain parts of the memory may not work as well as they might when being pounded with information and expected to come up with answers.

During the night the body manages to supply enough sugar to the brain to keep it going by calling on supplies. By the time the morning comes, energy requirements shoot up. Muscles used for getting out of bed, getting dressed and finally rushing out of the door and heading for school need to be refuelled. This means that, on rising, there is a possible relative shortage of sugar getting to the brain. This matters, because blood-sugar levels regulate a variety of brain functions, including learning and memory.

Memory is an amazing thing. Think back to when you last went into a supermarket. You probably wandered around getting all your usual things. If somebody asked you where a fancy display of baked beans was, you probably couldn't remember. However, if you had knocked those baked beans over, you'd remember exactly where they were. Not only that, you would remember what some of the people who stood and gawped looked like, as well as the furious face of the employee who had to pick up all the cans. The memory would be indelibly printed on your brain in the same way that many adults can remember exactly where they were, who they were with and what they were doing over three decades ago when they heard the news that President Kennedy had been shot. People will have similarly vivid memories associated with hearing the tragic news about Princess Diana.

This indelible printing is apparently stimulated by a rush of glucose to the brain at the time of the shock. This is caused by the release of the hormone adrenaline, which surges around your body at times like these. If the level of glucose in your brain can have such a profound effect on these kinds of memory, it's possible to see that smaller fluctuations may also have an effect on memory and brain functioning. Of course, this doesn't just go for children, but for adults too. If you have a demanding job that requires concentration for operating machinery or working at a desk, or have important decisions to make or tricky meetings to get through, having your memory and concentration skills in peak condition is crucial for your success as well.

Where's the Proof?

Many tests have been done on children to get to the bottom of the idea that skipping breakfast could bring their school performance down. Some researchers have discovered in laboratory settings that children who eat breakfast score better in tests which involve matching up familiar figures. Eating breakfast has also been shown to have beneficial effects on reaction times and problem solving, especially in children who have lower IQs. In other tests, researchers have seen improved scores in maths tasks.

The evidence is by no means 100 per cent conclusive and it does not show that having breakfast affects all facets of memory skill and related school work. However, much of the evidence is very interesting and suggests that it may be possible to optimize your children's potential. A study carried out on children in third world countries who were poorly nourished revealed that they were able to speak more fluently after having a breakfast which supplied a quarter of their day's food requirements.

In the Boardroom

Work carried out on adults in Wales showed that having breakfast improved their 'free recall' ability. Each person was shown a list of twenty words at a rate of one every two seconds. At the end, the subject had two minutes to write down the words in any order. Those who had eaten breakfast did better than those who had not.

Breakfast-eaters also did better at the 'delayed recognition memory task'. This was carried out at the end of the free-recall test. The adults were shown forty words. Twenty were the ones in the previous test, and twenty were added to distract them. Participants had to decide as quickly as possible which words had been shown in the original list.

From the Laboratory to the Classroom

These tests, on both children and adults, were carried out in scientific laboratories. Those taking part knew that their food was being altered and that the tests were taking place. A British researcher, Dr David Wyon, decided to put the 'breakfast improves performance' theory to the test in a school environment, and to change the type of breakfast the children ate at home. The children thought their breakfasts were being altered as part of a market research campaign, not because of tests that would later be carried out on them in school. He and his team carried out the study on almost two hundred ten-year-old children, attending five different schools in Sweden.

Two breakfasts were used in the research. One supplied a maximum of 197 calories for boys and 147 calories for girls, and consisted of a fresh bread roll, some low-fat margarine, diet raspberry jam and diet orange cordial. The other supplied 832 calories for boys and 567 calories for girls, and consisted of Corn Flakes, milk, an apple, fresh bread rolls, low-fat margarine, processed soft cheese, a slice of ham and a glass of orange juice. The children were allowed to eat as much or as little as they wanted from each breakfast, but unknown to them, their parents were measuring what was left. It was worked out that on average boys ate 563 calories from the big breakfast, while girls ate 434. With the small breakfast boys ate 170 calories while girls ate 121.

Tests in addition, multiplication, grammatical reasoning, number checking and creativity were carried out during normal lessons. The day after the tests the children also answered a questionnaire which asked them about how they had felt during the previous morning. For example, were they hungry before lunchtime? What sort of lunch did they have?

As well as the academic tests, the children also took part in their regular gym class, where physical endurance was measured. Just before lunch on the last day of the experiment their teachers asked them to fill out a form detailing how they felt. Do you feel good/bad? Do you have a headache/no headache? Feel giddy/not giddy?, and so on.

The results were interesting. When it came to both creativity and voluntary physical endurance, the effects of the higher-energy breakfast were found to be positive and significant. Ability to perform the addition and number-checking tests also *improved* in the children who ate *most* from the lower-energy breakfast compared to those who ate least from this choice.

Both boys and girls felt more hungry after the smaller breakfast, and it's not hard to imagine how that gnawing feeling in the pit of your stomach could put you off concentrating on what a teacher is saying. More children reported feeling bad rather than good during the morning when they'd eaten the smaller breakfast.

Dr Wyon came up with a pretty firm statement following the publication of his work:

'I think that parents who don't make sure that children have eaten a good breakfast before school are, in effect, handicapping them in their school work in several different ways. Our studies show that children's school performance is affected by their nutritional status in the very short term. Therefore, it is important that children are fed breakfast in some way. There are far too many people who skip breakfast; we know that from various studies in developed countries.'

Does it Matter what you Eat?

David Wyon's research showed clearly that the higher-energy breakfast outshone the lower-energy breakfast. Dr David Benton works in the Department of Psychology at the University of Wales in Swansea. He has also looked into the role of breakfast in improving performance, specifically the effects breakfast has on raising blood-sugar levels. He found that his human guinea pigs had an improved capacity to recall words in a test when they had eaten breakfast, and were able to remember more from a story that was read aloud to them. He also found, however, that their scores in intelligence tests were unaffected.

Benton explains that although the brain accounts for only 2 per cent of the body's weight, it uses up around 20–30 per cent of the body's total energy requirements. The amount of sugar or energy it is able to store is very small and without replacement would be exhausted in under ten minutes. It has always been assumed that the body keeps the brain optimally supplied with sugar almost at the expense of every other organ. This idea is now being challenged with the findings that improving blood sugar, through for example the simple task of eating breakfast after the night's fast, raises blood glucose and improves performance.

So does this mean that sucking a sweet or taking a sugar drink will have just as much effect as eating a balanced meal at breakfast? The answer is probably no, since Benton has found that a balanced meal improves recall better than a sugar hit. It is possible, therefore, that the other nutrients provided by breakfast are also playing a role in improving memory.

The precise ways in which blood-sugar levels affect the memory banks are not fully understood, but some mechanisms have been established. For example, blood sugar increases the production of a nerve transmitter called acetylcholine. Drugs that block this transmitter have been shown to disrupt memory, in particular reducing the ability to remember new information. Blood sugar needs vitamin B1 (thiamin) to make acetylcholine.

Benton writes: 'It is possible that the development of food items that both offer an optimal supply of glucose and improve the micro-nutrient status to allow its utilization, may benefit cognition . . . Breakfast products that are based on cereal and are fortified with various micro-nutrients offer one such approach.'

Your Questions Answered

I've only got time to give the girls toast before we all rush out in the morning. Is this OK?

Anything is better than nothing, but regularly consuming fortified cereals at breakfast has the advantage of supplying the body with extra iron and other vital minerals and vitamins. Studies have found that teenage girls who are on the border of iron deficiency can improve their performance in IQ tests by 9 points (the difference between a D and C grade in GCSEs) by upping their iron intakes. Anaemia caused through a lack of iron leads to tiredness and inability to concentrate – hardly the symptoms you want to handicap your children with at school. If they can fit in a bowl of fortified breakfast cereal before their toast you could be helping them reach their full potential at school.

My daughter and son just refuse to eat breakfast. They say they're not hungry. Is there anything I can do?

Take a two-pronged approach. First, take a look at what time they eat their evening meal. If it's late, then bring it forward. The later they eat the less hungry they will feel on waking. The same is true if they are overtired. So, secondly, check how much sleep they are getting. If they are tired in the mornings, not only will they lie in for as long as possible, thus sacrificing breakfasting time, they also probably won't feel hungry once they've dragged their sleepy selves out of bed. Children eat bigger breakfasts during the school holidays, probably because they have more time and are less tired. Set some new habits in place for the term time. You could be improving their future school results.

The National Breakfast Week Schools Campaign

In 1997 lots of teachers throughout the country took up the challenge to raise their pupils' awareness of the importance of eating breakfast before leaving home, and to tell them how this simple daily habit could help in the classroom. From Perthshire to Glamorgan, from Sheffield to Essex, teachers set up posters, gave out leaflets and supplied pupils with packets of cereal. This is what a few of them had to say about the week's activities:

Pat Frazier Greening, Deputy Head Teacher, Aston Tower Junior School, Birmingham

'I displayed the posters supplied around the school and took an assembly telling the children about the benefits of breakfast.

The first thing I had to do was to admit to them that, before reading the information, I normally didn't have breakfast myself! I told them what I'd started to eat and suggested that they try cereals, toast and fruit, and that eating something like this could help them do better at school. During the week I stopped children in the corridors and asked them if they'd had breakfast that day. It's surprising just how many don't have anything to eat before leaving home and the first thing they eat is at break-time when half the morning's lessons have gone. We gave them some individual packets of cereals and asked them to try to have them during the week. I told them that eating breakfast had made me feel much better and gave me more energy. Hopefully some of them listened and tried to leave time for breakfast.'

Schools Nurse, south-east Belfast

'We set up our breakfast promotion week in a grammar school in south-east Belfast. Our stand was right by the reception and in addition to the posters and leaflets we cooked toast and brewed coffee to attract the pupils' interest. A small survey we conducted over the week showed that lots of kids are coming to school without breakfast, often because both of their parents are working and they rush to drop the children off to school so that they can get to work. We were so surprised by this that the school decided to start up a breakfast club so that children could get something to eat before school started.'

Liz Mitchell, teacher at Falkirk High School, Falkirk

'We missed National Breakfast Week last year but have decided to make use of the pack of information in the summer over our two- to three-day induction period when we welcome new children to the school. A large proportion of children seem to come to school without eating any breakfast so we'd like them to understand how important it is to try to make time for it. It would be great if we could set up a breakfast club in school. It would benefit them because they would learn more, and it would benefit the school because they'd be able to concentrate more. Of course the problem is it is expensive to set this kind of club up. Sadly the money's just not there. Hopefully though we will encourage them to have breakfast before leaving home.'

Ann Vinters, Marks Gate Infants School, Essex

'We've been involved for two years now with Kellogg's National Breakfast Week and the children really enjoy it. We talk to them about why they should eat breakfast and give them individual packets of cereal to take home which they are thrilled with. Lots of our children do miss breakfast, while others come in just eating a packet of crisps. By lunchtime they are really quite hungry. I worry about those who miss breakfast, especially with the new literacy and numeracy hours which are being introduced, which require the children to concentrate hard for these two hours. Without breakfast inside of them, they could find it very difficult.'

And Finally Breakfast – A Great Natural De-Stresser

Do you always wake up feeling you've got out of bed the wrong side? Never feel good until lunchtime? Maybe fuelling up before you leave home could get your day off to a brighter start. Although there has not been a lot of research into the area of breakfast and mood, it is possible to conclude from work which has been done that a low-fat, high-carbohydrate breakfast like cereal with low-fat milk leads to improved mood in the morning.

Such a meal has also been found to make people feel less tired, dreamy and weak than when they had a high-fat, low-carbohydrate breakfast. Finally, in tests on old people, breakfast has been shown to make those studied feel more calm and less tense.

Chapter 6

How a Vitamin in your Breakfast may help prevent Heart Disease

There can't be many people around today who haven't heard of the word cholesterol or don't know that it's got something to do with heart disease. For years scientists have been uncovering its role in the development of one of our country's biggest killer diseases. They have told us over and over again to cut down on fat, especially saturated animal fat, in order to help keep cholesterol levels down. Now the world of medical research is coming up with some exciting new ideas about how our food may help in our battle to reduce heart disease.

It has been said that this new dietary approach may one day prove to be as important as decreasing blood pressure, lowering cholesterol and giving up smoking in reducing our risk of developing heart disease.

If that sounds like good news, wait until you hear this. For once we are not being told to reduce foods we currently love tucking into, but instead are being encouraged to eat more of something. If that's not a breakthrough I don't know what is. And what should we be eating more of? A little-heard-of vitamin, belonging to the B group, called 'folic acid'.

Although we may have heard little of it, some scientists have been working on the theory that folic acid and several other B vitamins could help in the prevention of heart disease for almost as long as those who've been looking into the cholesterol story. Indeed the folic acid saga began nearly thirty years ago with an outstanding American pathologist called Dr Kilmer McCully.

Now 63, McCully has dedicated almost his entire working life to the theory that folic acid levels in our diets may affect our chances of having heart disease. Like so many great discoveries, it started with a hunch. He became intrigued by two children who had died from a rare genetic disease called homocystinuria. People with this disease have raised levels of a substance called homocysteine (pronounced ho-mo-SIS-teen) in their blood. As well as having severe learning difficulties, many people with this disease tragically never live past their mid-teens, in most cases dying with severely ravaged arteries that have been clogged by the process known as atherosclerosis.

On examining the arteries of these two children, McCully saw that their blood vessels had lost elasticity and were narrowed to the extent you usually see in elderly people. He began to realize that perhaps it was the high levels of homocysteine in the blood that had directly damaged the cells and tissues of the arteries, in much the same way that cholesterol was, at the time, thought to do. Certainly, experiments carried out in test-tubes suggested this to be the case, with homocysteine injuring blood-vessel linings and accelerating the build-up of scar tissue that leads to blood clots.

Homocystinuria, however, is a rare genetic problem. The question McCully had to ask was how his theory could affect the rest of us. While full-blown homocystinuria is indeed rare, McCully predicted that even people with very small increases in blood homocysteine could be affected. That could mean many hundreds of thousands of the population at large. As his work progressed, this extraordinary scientist looked for reasons why small increases in homocysteine might occur and how they could be lowered, questions which led him to folic acid and two other B vitamins.

B Vitamins and Homocysteine Levels

To understand the role of B vitamins and homocysteine, you need to know where homocysteine comes from, and how levels are normally kept very tightly controlled within a tiny range. So here goes. Homocysteine isn't found in foods in the way, for example, vitamin C or the mineral iron is. Instead, the body forms it by breaking down a protein substance known as methionine. Methionine is found in large amounts in protein foods such as meat, eggs and milk. In the body, it is broken down into homocysteine, which is used for doing quick repair jobs, building and maintaining surrounding tissues. Homocysteine is not meant to hang around for long, however, and is normally either quickly broken down into other complicated substances or made back into methionine. These breakdown processes are controlled by enzymes (substances that start up and control the speed of many processes in the body). These enzymes must have folic acid, B6 and B12 in order to work properly. McCully became fascinated with the idea that if homocysteine levels were raised, it was because these enzymes were not working properly and that this malfunction could be due to a lack of these vitamins in the diet.

In other words, homocysteine levels could be higher when intakes of B vitamins were low.

McCully wondered whether by increasing these B vitamins he could get homocysteine levels to fall. He tested his theory on animals with high homocysteine – and bingo. Within hours of giving them these vitamins, levels started to fall. Once he was convinced of the link, he and others started testing it on humans.

As you can imagine, this kind of research requires large sums of money to fund. Sadly, in spite of the exciting results that McCully and others were getting, in the mid-1970s the cholesterol story was the more trendy of the two. Scientists working in the cholesterol area attracted the cash, while McCully's theory was left in the scientific wastelands. The folic acid–homocysteine theory was put on ice.

The big Melt

As with previous ice ages, the big melt eventually came. It was some fifteen years later that other enlightened researchers in the United States, Ireland, Sweden, Norway and the Netherlands began to take an interest in McCully's ideas. By 1990 some of these findings began to arouse the interest of the scientific world, and with interest, came cash. The coffers of the funders once again opened. This coincided with the understanding that, while blood cholesterol is an important part of the jigsaw in the development of heart disease, it's not the only diet-related factor.

The Story unfolds

To give the folic acid and homocysteine theory credibility, it needed more heavyweights in the scientific world to take it seriously. This started to happen in 1992, when an important professor at Harvard School of Public Health in the United States took a look at blood samples collected decades earlier from 271 doctors as part of a large study into long-term diseases. They had all been healthy at the time they gave their blood. Professor Stampfer found that those who had gone on to have myocardial infarction (where the heart muscle doesn't get enough blood) had, in many cases, higher levels of homocysteine in their blood than those who remained fit. The levels were not outrageously high, and were nothing like as raised as in people with homocystinuria, but even so, those with the highest levels had the greatest chance of developing heart disease.

A Norwegian scientist called Arnesen made similar findings three years later in 1995. Of 20,000 apparently healthy people who gave blood, 123 had gone on to develop heart disease. Again, the levels of homocysteine in their blood samples were found to be higher than those who had not developed heart disease. Many other studies revealed similar findings, while another showed there also to be a link between raised homocysteine and stroke. The story was looking exciting and this time round was attracting lots more interest.

Folic Acid taken Seriously

It is now established that McCully had the right idea. Folic acid and other B vitamins control the working of the enzymes that remove homocysteine from the blood, and it seems that raised homocysteine does play an important role in the development of heart disease. It's been found both that people with heart disease often have higher levels of homocysteine, and that apparently healthy people who had higher levels in their blood had subsequently a higher risk of dying of heart disease than those with lower levels.

Not just the Men

While a lot of the work on homocysteine and heart disease has dealt with men, some has dealt with women, which is just as well since the British Heart Foundation tells us that 1 in 5 women in the UK die of heart disease. This is important – we often think of heart disease as a 'man's problem', in the same way that PMS is a 'woman's problem'. This recent study on women looked back at the dietary intake of a huge group of American nurses and found an association between high intakes of folic acid and a lower incidence of heart disease. Back in 1980, over 80,000 samples of blood were taken from these women who, at the same time as giving their blood, also completed questionnaires about their diet. All were free from heart disease at the time of giving blood. Fourteen years later 658 were found to have non-fatal myocardial infarctions (where some of the heart muscle doesn't get enough blood and oxygen) and 281 had actually died of heart disease. When their dietary records were looked at, sure enough, those who had eaten breakfast cereals fortified with folic acid or those who had taken supplements had the highest intake of folic acid and a lower incidence of heart disease.

Is Folic Acid more important than B6 and B12?

All three are needed to control the breakdown and subsequent removal of homocysteine from the blood. A shortage of any of these will lead to raised homocysteine. The fact is very few of us don't eat enough B6 and B12, although as far as B12 is concerned, if there is a problem, it's more likely to be absorption than intake. Very strict vegans may not get enough if they don't eat foods fortified with B12 or take supplements.

With folic acid it's not so simple. Folic acid is the name given to the synthetic version of the vitamin folate. Folate is found in dark green vegetables such as spinach, Brussels sprouts and in wholegrain foods such as wholemeal bread.

The trouble is, even if you are eating these kinds of foods regularly (and, let's face it, how many of us do?), the body finds it quite hard to absorb the folate. It's thought that around half the folate eaten doesn't make it into the bloodstream. Professor John Scott and his research group are based at Trinity College, Dublin. They are leading lights in the field of folic acid and homocysteine research and have shown, in a study carried out in 1996, just how hard it is for folate in foods to raise blood folate levels.

They divided a group of sixty-two women into five smaller groups.

Group 1 had to try to eat 400 micrograms of folate-rich foods such as Brussels sprouts and spinach a day.

Group 2 were given foods fortified with the synthetic version of folate (in other words, foods fortified with folic acid, such as breakfast cereals). Again, 400 micrograms a day was the target.

Group 3 took a 400 microgram folic acid supplement daily.

Group 4 were given *advice* on how to increase their intake of folate-rich foods to supply 400 micrograms a day.

Group 5 were given no special foods and no advice – they were the control group against which the others were to be measured.

Their results revealed that levels of folate in the blood only increased significantly in the women who ate foods fortified with folic acid and those taking the folic acid supplements. This suggested that you could tell people until you were blue in the face how to up their folate naturally, and even make them eat lots of folate-rich foods, but this would make very little difference to their overall blood-folate levels or body stores of folate. Get them to eat folic acid-enriched foods or pop a supplement on the other hand, and Bob's your uncle: up go the blood levels of folate and, hopefully, if you suffer with raised homocysteine levels, down they come.

Can taking Folic Acid lower Homocysteine?

All of this research was vital. The next step was to determine scientifically whether by increasing folic acid intake in a group of apparently healthy people, homocysteine levels could be reduced, and then to find out over time whether these people had a reduced risk of dying of heart disease. These are the million-dollar questions that have started to be answered by the likes, among others, of Professor Scott and his team in Ireland.

In one experiment Scott and his team took a group of thirty healthy men and gave them folic acid supplements for 26 weeks. One group had 100 micrograms a day, another 200 micrograms and the third 400 micrograms. Blood samples were taken before, during, and at ten weeks after the supplementation had stopped. Blood levels of folate and homocysteine were measured. Of the three folic acid doses given, 200 micrograms and 400 micrograms were found to be the most effective at lowering homocysteine. The results led the scientists to conclude that a daily dose of 200 micrograms of folic acid is effective in lowering homocysteine in regular, everyday people who seem outwardly to be a picture of health.

The Future – does reducing Homocysteine reduce Heart Disease?

More and larger studies need to be carried out to establish this connection conclusively and to see if heart-disease rates are reduced over time. Many scientists feel that 200 micrograms (and some say even 100) of extra folic acid a day may be enough for optimal reduction of blood homocysteine in the population as a whole. The medical world seems broadly to agree that the idea – that small increases of folic acid in our diets may reduce heart disease – is looking powerful. So convinced are the Americans of this link that many believe that the government's order that all flour, pasta, rice, noodles and corn grits be fortified with folic acid could lead to a decrease in future rates of heart disease as well as of spina bifida, which was the main reason for its being added in the first place. You can read more about this fortification scheme in Chapter 7.

How many of us have raised Homocysteine?

It was McCully who first asked the question: if severe increases in homocysteine in children with homocystinuria can destroy their arteries, could milder but longer-term increases be damaging to people without this disease? It seems likely that our diet and lifestyle can affect our homocysteine levels. A low intake of the vital B vitamins can affect levels, and it's been shown that other risk factors such as lack of exercise, ageing and smoking also raise homocysteine. Men appear to have naturally higher levels than women. It is also now believed that about one in eight of us inherits a gene that slows down the removal of homocysteine from our blood, leaving us with higher than desirable levels. It's possible that raised homocysteine accounts for some of the sudden deaths from heart disease that occur among young and seemingly fit people.

At the moment no quick, cheap tests are available for measuring homocysteine, but this isn't a huge issue for the general public since, unlike cholesterol, there is no definite figure above which you are more at risk of heart disease. Instead it seems to be a graded response, with increasing risk across a full range of homocysteine levels. It is estimated that up to 60 per cent of us could reduce our homocysteine levels by increasing folic acid intakes.

Should we Increase our Intakes of Folate and Folic Acid?

In the United Kingdom, population studies have revealed that the average intake of folate is around 200 micrograms a day. This is the recommended intake the government suggested back in 1991. However, since 1991 the government has recommended that women who are trying to become pregnant should increase this by a further 400 micrograms a day (to 600 micrograms) to reduce the risk of having a baby with spina bifida (see Chapter 7).

Furthermore, it would appear from studies that increasing intake of both folic acid and folates in the general population may keep the homocysteine levels on the low rather than high side of normal. The United States has taken a dramatic step in this direction. In January 1998 their Food and Drug Administration passed the law that folic acid was to be added to flour, rice, noodles and corn grits. In other words bread, cakes and pasta, to mention a few commonly consumed cereal-based foods, now contain added folic acid.

The decision to fortify these common grains was encouraged by work carried out by an American called Carol Boushey. Boushey rounded up the results of thirty-eight studies looking into folic acid and homocysteine, and concluded that by adding 140 micrograms of folic acid to every 100 grams of grain, it may be possible to prevent around 7 per cent of fatal male heart disease and 5 per cent of female coronary-related deaths. On the basis of Boushey's conclusions, which took into account many other scientists' work in this area, it was decided that, in spite of absence of absolute proof, fortification could go ahead.

This decision was taken primarily to help reduce the number of babies born with spina bifida, but the potential reduction this could bring to homocysteine levels and thus possibly to heart disease was considered an added incentive. The result of fortification is that American intakes of folate and folic acid have jumped on average from 200 to 300 micrograms a day.

How can we improve Intakes here?

As yet the UK government hasn't agreed to blanket fortification of a staple food with folic acid. Improving our intakes is therefore down to us. In what you eat, it's worth increasing both foods fortified with folic acid, and foods that naturally contain folate since they, besides improving blood levels a little, are inherently healthy foods that supply a whole host of other vital nutrients.

Spinach, for example, has folate but also supplies us with vitamin E, the minerals iron and calcium, plus some fibre. Wholemeal bread has folate but is also rich in fibre and energy-releasing B vitamins, and oranges supply not just folate but lots of vitamin C. Of course you can also take a daily supplement of folic acid to boost intakes.

To date, fortification with folic acid by food manufacturers here in the UK is voluntary. If you shop wisely, however, you can find products whose manufacturers have decided to add extra folic acid. Breakfast cereals are one such example. Tests have shown that eating these cereals raises blood folate levels and body stores of folate. When the cereals were removed from the diet, blood folate levels fell. Wholemeal bread fortified with folic acid is another example: it then contains both naturally occurring folate and added folic acid.

The Folic Acid Flash

In 1997 the Health Education Authority backed a labelling initiative which sets out to show clearly if folic acid has been added to a product. The distinctive blue circle around the letter 'F' can be found on certain fortified breakfast cereals and breads.

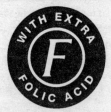

Products using this claim supply around 100 micrograms of folic acid per serving. These include:

ASDA Milk for Women
ASDA Yeast Extract
Kellogg's Rice Krispies
Kellogg's Corn Flakes

Kellogg's Special K

Marmite and Bovril

Mighty White medium and Mighty White thick sliced bread

Sainsbury's white medium-sliced bread, soft-grain medium-sliced bread and soft-grain thick-sliced bread

Sainsbury's Yeast Extract

Tesco Healthy Eating white bread, Healthy Eating wholemeal bread and soft grain bread

Village Bakery: Harvester sliced, Village sliced and most other loaves, fruit scones and tea cakes, bara brith and barm cakes

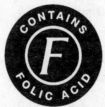

'Contains Folic Acid' means the food supplies us with at least 33 micrograms of folic acid per average portion. Such foods include:

Kellogg's: Healthwise Bran Flakes, Healthwise Sultana Bran, All-Bran Plus, Sustain, Raisin Wheats, Choco Corn Flakes, Country Store, Multi-Grain Start, Just Right, All-Bran Bite Size, Optima Fruit and Fibre, Choco Krispies, All-Bran Buds, Bran Buds, Common Sense, Apple Wheats, Frosties, Frosted Wheat, Nut Feast, Corn Pops, Honey Loops, Strike, Ricicles, Crunchy Nut Corn Flakes

Mother's Pride: Champion thick-sliced and medium-sliced

Nestlé: Build-up strawberry, chocolate, lemon and lime and natural drinks, plus potato and leek, and chicken- and mushroom-flavoured soups

MD Foods: Bio-Yoghurt

Folate in Foods

RICH SOURCES: More than 100 micrograms per serving
Fresh, raw or cooked (10–20 minutes) Brussels sprouts, aspar-
agus, spinach, kale; cooked black-eye beans

GOOD SOURCES: 50–100 micrograms per serving
Fresh, raw, frozen and cooked (10–20 minutes) broccoli, spring
greens, cabbage, green beans, cauliflower, peas, beansprouts,
okra, cooked soya beans, iceberg lettuce, parsnips, chickpeas
(large portions of broccoli, cauliflower and spring greens will
supply more than 100 micrograms)
Kidneys, and yeast and beef extracts

MODERATE SOURCES: 15–50 micrograms per serving
Potatoes, most other fresh and cooked vegetables, most fruits,
most nuts and tahini
Bread (100 grams), brown rice, wholegrain pasta, oats, bran
Cheese, yoghurt, milk (1 pint/568 ml), eggs, salmon, beef, game

POOR SOURCES: Less than 15 micrograms per serving
White rice, white pasta, alcoholic drinks, soft drinks, sugar,
most pastries, cakes, most other meats and fish
Most other breakfast cereals (not fortified with folic acid)

Note: Pregnant women and those intending to become pregnant
are advised not to eat liver or liver products because of the risk
of possible adverse effects from consuming excess vitamin A.

Can you eat too much Folic Acid?

It is possible that very large intakes of folic acid – say around
5,000 micrograms a day taken in supplement form – may mask
the presence of a type of anaemia caused by lack of vitamin B12.
It was suggested by Carol Boushey that anyone taking supplements of 4,000 micrograms of folic acid should also take 1

milligram of vitamin B12, thereby correcting any B12 deficiencies and considerably lessening the concern over the masking effects of folic acid.

Folic Acid – a Simple Solution for a Mammoth Problem?

Many people now feel that fortifying foods with folic acid could help slash the number of heart attack cases in Britain. Given that diseases of the heart and cardiovascular system are still one of our country's biggest killers, claiming some 300,000 deaths in 1995 and costing the NHS a massive £1,600 million a year, anything we can do to decrease these numbers must be worth a try. We know we should be taking care about raised cholesterol and blood pressure. We know we should stop smoking. Most of us realize that being overweight increases the risk of heart disease too. How many of us realize that simply by improving intakes of folic acid yet more deaths may also be avoided? You can help yourself, and your family and friends, by looking for, buying and regularly eating foods with the folic acid flash.

Heart Disease and Cholesterol

Reducing your intake of animal fats can help in the bid to lower blood cholesterol levels. Cutting back on fatty cuts of meat, reducing the amount of butter and full-fat dairy foods you eat and keeping a strict eye on cakes and biscuits are all ways of achieving this. You will notice that all of these changes to your diet involve reducing or cutting back. Here's some better news. Regularly eating breakfast seems to help reduce cholesterol levels.

Regularly eating breakfast may help to reduce your risk of heart disease not just because it's an easy meal at which to raise your folic acid intake, but also because starting the day with the right kind of meal can also help to lower blood cholesterol. This has been shown to be the case in quite a few studies. One that looked at a group of almost 200 nine to nineteen-year-olds showed that even in these young people cholesterol was lowest in those who ate a cereal breakfast (especially one high in dietary fibre), and highest in those who skipped it or who feasted on a high-fat meal.

In another test of almost 12,000 people, it was again revealed that breakfast skippers had the highest cholesterol. Still more work on over a thousand people ranging in age from just two through to ninety-seven showed that high intakes of breakfast cereals were associated with lower serum cholesterol levels. It's not firmly established that the people with lower cholesterol levels had lower rates of heart disease, because the studies didn't go on for long enough. But we do know that, in general, raised cholesterol – like smoking, being overweight and having raised blood pressure – does make you more prone to heart problems.

It's possible that this cholesterol-lowering effect of eating breakfast, especially a cereal breakfast, has something to do with the fact that it tends to reduce the overall amount of fat we eat. By reducing the total amount of fat, we reduce saturated fat, which could help bring cholesterol down. Not only this, it could help reduce our weight, which might also help protect against heart disease.

Chapter 7

How a Simple B Vitamin may help prevent Spina Bifida

As a baby is growing in the womb, one of the very first parts of its body to develop is something called the neural tube. Dr Chris Schorah, Senior Fellow at the University of Leeds, explains. 'The neural tube starts off as a plate of nerve cells which rolls over onto itself to create a tube. This goes on to become the spine. The process happens very early on in pregnancy, around days twenty to twenty-eight. If the nerve material doesn't fuse into a tube all the way down then a so-called neural tube defect occurs.'

If this fusion fails at what becomes the bottom of the spine, the condition called spina bifida results. All this is happening way before most women have the faintest notion they are pregnant. Spina bifida affects babies in different ways, but depending on its severity can mean a future of dependence on other people and being unable to walk or control the bladder. Some very extreme forms of neural tube defects mean the baby cannot survive.

Every day in England and Wales, at least two babies are conceived with neural tube defects such as spina bifida. Of the 750,000-plus births in the UK each year, neural tube problems occur in almost 400. A further 1,600 pregnancies are affected, resulting either in termination or stillbirth. Potentially, everyone's baby is at risk, whatever your age, whether you have other children, and even if spina bifida has never appeared in your family.

It has now been shown that the level of the B vitamin folate in the blood of certain women somehow affects the closing of the neural tube. Increasing folate levels in the blood through increasing the amount of naturally occurring folate-rich foods in the diet is hard because folate is not very well absorbed in the body and much of it is lost on cooking and storage. Eating foods fortified with the synthetic form, folic acid, and taking supplements of folic acid is believed to be the most effective way to guarantee increased blood folate levels. (This is covered in more detail in Chapter 6.)

It has been shown in research that mothers who have already had one child with spina bifida can drastically reduce the risk of having another baby with the same condition by eating folic acid-enriched foods or taking supplements. In addition, it is believed that eating more folic acid can help prevent women having a first child with spina bifida.

How the Link was Discovered

Controversy over the relationship between folic acid and neural tube defects had, like the link between folic acid, homocysteine and heart disease, been raging for some three decades.

Evidence that intakes of folate and folic acid may play a crucial role in preventing spina bifida had been mounting since the 1960s, but it wasn't until July 1991, when the Medical Research Council reported convincing results on its protective effects, that things started to become clear. Their research involved 1,817 women, each of whom had had a baby with a neural tube defect. Of the 1,195 women who became pregnant, twenty-seven gave birth to babies with a neural tube defect. Twenty-one of these were born to mothers who had not taken folic acid, and only six to those who had. These results suggested that taking folic acid supplements would give the women a staggering 72 per cent rate of protection against having a second child with spina bifida.

As a result of this research, the government took the unusual step of recommending that all women who had had a child with spina bifida should take a 4 milligram supplement of folic acid every day if they were trying for another baby. Women like Therese, who's forty-one and comes from Tamworth in Staffordshire. Therese heard about this news very soon after it was released in late 1991. She explains:

'I had already had two healthy sons when I heard about folic acid and by this stage I was pregnant with Samantha, who, I was told at my sixteen-week scan, had spina bifida. They put me on supplements of 4 milligrams a day which I kept taking for two or three months after Samantha was born. It was already too late to change Samantha's condition but it turned out that taking the folic acid must have been the right thing to do because quite out of the blue I became pregnant again just nine months later and gave birth to Catherine who was completely healthy. There's a much higher chance of having a second baby with spina bifida after you have had a first one, and in my mind it was the folic acid I took during and after Sam's pregnancy that protected Catherine.'

How Important is Folic Acid for Women of Childbearing Age?

The advice covered women who were known to be at high risk of having children with neural tube problems. What about the rest of the women in the country who may have a baby in the future? After all, over 95 per cent of neural tube defects are first occurrences. In other words, either a first-born, or born to mothers whose previous children had not had spina bifida.

Most women and men in this country are currently eating around 200 micrograms of folic acid a day in the form of natural folates from foods such as fruit and vegetables and wholemeal bread. The government felt that the best advice they could give to women previously unaffected with a spina bifida baby who were planning a pregnancy was to increase their intake of folic acid by a further 400 micrograms a day. This would make a regular daily total of some 600 micrograms.

Therese comments: 'All women who are of an age when they might become pregnant, even if they aren't planning it, should take a 400-microgram-a-day supplement, as well as eating a good diet and including foods which bear the folic acid flash. I'm lobbying my MP to get folic acid added to flour. I say to him, if they put it in Corn Flakes for heaven's sake it must be safe. By increasing everyone's intakes in this way you would reach the girls and women who get pregnant by accident. As far as the folic acid flashes go, I think they are great, but manufacturers need to be able to advertise the reasons why folic acid has been added. At the moment they are not allowed to do so. It needs to be on the adverts in between Coronation Street, that's where the message would get through.

'We adore and love Sam so much. She's given us back a million times what we've given her. But she does have to cope with a lot just to get through every day. It takes us two hours to get her ready for school, what with doing physio' and sorting out her catheters. She has to see four consultants, which means on average she has fortnightly visits to the hospital. She has to use a wheelchair for much of the time. I'm enormously proud of all her achievements but if the risk of this disease can be reduced by taking more of a simple B vitamin called folic acid, then everyone has the right to know about it.'

Kate, a Mum from Chester who has a five-year-old son with spina bifida, agrees: 'I found out I was pregnant just over six years ago when I was thirty-two. At the time there was absolutely no publicity about folic acid and the need to take it before or during pregnancy. It's getting better but it's still not widely enough known. Since having Tom, who has spina bifida, I became aware of the issues and took folic acid supplements while trying to conceive again. My second son Toby is nearly three and healthy. I wouldn't want other people to go through what Tom and all of us as a family have been through. If you are thinking of getting pregnant, or even if you're not, all I can say is for goodness sake take supplements and eat foods rich in folic acid which bear the With Extra Folic Acid mark, like fortified breakfast cereals and bread.'

For sources of folate and folic acid, see page 48.

How Folic Acid may work against Spina Bifida

Scientists don't always have all the answers, and this is one of the cases where they don't. They know there is a relationship between increasing folic acid intakes and preventing spina bifida, but they aren't absolutely sure what the relationship is. It could be that taking extra folic acid corrects a deficiency where the woman isn't eating enough folate, or where what she is eating isn't being absorbed well. It could also be that the woman has a metabolic blockage, a bit like a clogged drain, where a bit of the folate gets through but not all. By loading the system with extra, more in total gets through.

Getting Enough Folic Acid

You could in theory boost folate by eating an extra portion of, say, Brussels sprouts, spinach and potatoes. In practice it's not so simple. Although these foods together would supply your 200 micrograms of folate, only around half of this gets absorbed. While no one should be discouraged from eating more foods naturally rich in folate (they also supply lots of other essential nutrients), there is a good argument for including more foods which have been fortified with the easily absorbed synthetic version – folic acid. Women actively trying to get pregnant should also take a 400 microgram supplement daily.

The Difference between Folate and Folic Acid

Folates, which are naturally present in the foods shown in the table on page 50, are vulnerable to heat and dissolve in water. Cooking may reduce levels before you get the foods on to your plate. Storage also depletes the natural folates in vegetables. The measured content of folates in food is, therefore, often only an approximate measure of what you are getting. There is also concern that folates eaten in food do not raise blood folate as effectively as may have been expected. In a study by Professor

John Scott and his team in Ireland, published in the *Lancet* in March 1996, it was shown that, compared with supplements and foods fortified with folic acid, consuming extra folate in natural foods is a relatively ineffective way of improving levels in the blood.

Fortifying Foods

In the United States it has been law since January 1998 that 140 micrograms of folic acid is added to every 100 grams of grain, which includes breadmaking flour, rice, noodles and corn grits. This action should mean that, on average, folic acid intakes increase by 100 micrograms a day in the general population. It may not be high enough to maximize prevention of neural tube defects caused by low folate levels, but it is a step in the right direction. Although an extra 400 micrograms of folic acid is ideal for the majority of women, research published in the *Lancet* in December 1997 has shown that if the general population continuously take 100 micrograms extra through fortified food we will see an important decrease in neural tube defects.

In the UK it is still undecided whether to add folic acid to grains by law. At the moment fortification is up to the food manufacturer. To help us spot which foods are fortified, the Health Education Authority has joined forces with the food industry to devise a 'flash' or mark to show foods that have been fortified with folic acid (see page 48). The Folic Acid Flash is part of an integrated campaign run by the Health Education Authority aimed at increasing by at least 400 micrograms a day the average intakes of folates and folic acid in women who may become pregnant, from foods naturally containing folates, foods fortified with folic acid, and folic acid supplements.

At the time of the flash launch in 1997, Health Education Director Kathy Elliott explained: 'Our awareness research found that only 3 per cent of women aged sixteen to forty-five knew that breakfast cereals and bread fortified with folic acid were readily available. The flash scheme will enable women to boost their intake of this essential B vitamin by easily selecting fortified foods off the supermarket shelf.'

The impact of the flashes on the population's understanding of folic acid was hoped to be dramatic. Take fortified breakfast cereals for example. Over just a three-month period some millions of packs of these cereals sat on people's breakfast tables. The flash and the accompanying health message about folic acid could not fail to get through to a good proportion of people as they tucked into their morning bowl of cereal.

A 30-gram serving of 'Extra Folic Acid' cereal with semi-skimmed milk provides a good 100 micrograms of folic acid. Most supermarket chains now also stock own-label soft-grain bread fortified with folic acid. Two slices supply around 90 micrograms of folic acid. A breakfast of fortified cereal and toast could therefore supply 190 micrograms of folic acid each morning.

How Effective has the Health Education Authority Campaign been?

To assess how far their campaign has improved knowledge of folic acid, the Health Education Authority has questioned the public. To see what proportion of women already knew of the importance of folic acid, the survey asked: 'What should pregnant women, or women who may become pregnant, eat or take more of?'

In 1995 only 9 per cent of women in their childbearing years had been aware of the importance of folic acid in their diet before and during pregnancy. By 1997 this had increased to 39 per cent.

When prompted over a connection between folic acid and pregnancy, 51 per cent in 1995 said they had heard of it. By 1997 this figure had risen to 84 per cent.

There's a long way to go, but things are clearly looking up and the message is getting across.

The Health Education Authority points out that not all pregnancies are planned, so trying to increase folic acid intakes is not only relevant to women thinking about having a baby.

Kathy Elliott explains: 'We know that an estimated 30–50 per cent of pregnancies are unintended, so women who regularly eat fortified breads and breakfast cereals will have an increased level of folic acid if they become pregnant unexpectedly.'

The Health Education Authority reports that, since starting the Folic Acid campaign, the number of brands of loaf fortified with folic acid has increased from eight (in December 1995) to twenty (in December 1997). The majority of the biggest retailers now produce an own-label brand of white soft-grain fortified bread. The Association of Cereal Manufacturers says that in July 1996 101 breakfast cereals were reported to be fortified with folic acid. By December 1997 this had risen to 112. You need to look carefully for the flashes and check the nutritional panel. Levels vary from 60 to 333 micrograms per 100 grams. Check our list for those with the highest levels: see page 48.

The Three-pronged Folic Acid Attack

Many people feel that the three-pronged approach – increasing folic acid-fortified foods, increasing naturally folate-rich foods and taking a 400 microgram supplement each day – is the best way for women of childbearing age to give themselves maximum protection against unexpected neural tube defects in their unborn child. For women who have already had a baby with spina bifida, a 4 *milligram* a day supplement of folic acid should be taken, which can be obtained on prescription. For other women, the 400 microgram supplements are available from health food stores, pharmacies and most supermarkets. They are small, easy to take and you need only one a day. Many different brands are available so you have a choice.

Getting the Message Across to Young Girls
in North Nottinghamshire

In addition to the Health Education Authority's nationwide campaign, some people have been promoting folic acid locally.

Penny Spice is the Senior Health Promotions Specialist in North Nottinghamshire. She and the local community dietitian applied for a Health Education Authority grant in 1997 to promote the folic acid story to young people in their area. On winning a £1,000 grant, a multi-agency working group decided to organize breakfast events at local schools.

'We chose two secondary schools, one in Mansfield, the other in Kirkby-in-Ashfield. The local Co-op worked with us, generously supplying lots of folic acid-fortified breakfast cereals and the milk to go on the cereals, as well as wholemeal bread and orange juice. With the grant we were able to pay catering staff to help us serve the breakfasts and explain the message about folic acid. We also used displays and gave out literature to show how breakfast is an easy meal at which to increase folic acid intake. Folic acid aside, some teachers at the school told us they thought there was a real problem with children not eating breakfast and then finding it hard to concentrate in class. The days we did the breakfast club they said they noticed the children had more energy and focus in lessons. After we finished our breakfast days, we looked through information we'd gleaned and found that a lot of fourteen-year-old girls were missing breakfast to help them control their weight, something I found really worrying. On the positive side, we also discovered that our days had achieved their main purpose, which was to improve awareness about folic acid.'

Chapter 8

Fighting the Flab – how Cereals help

Few of us can have missed the continual tickings off we get from health experts on television, radio and in magazines over Britain's expanding waistline. It's true that as a nation we are getting larger, and if we don't take things in hand, it really is only going to be a matter of time before we end up like the Americans where over half the country is now obese. If you're not convinced then how about this. Boeing's aircraft designers have recently been forced to increase the assumed weight of each passenger by an astounding 20 pounds to ensure they can still get off the ground and stay airborne. Weight is climbing countrywide, and at the moment Walsall comes out at the top of the table for fatness in the UK, a city which has, appropriately enough, a sculpture of a hippopotamus at its centre.

In Walsall they have a passion for such local delicacies as Desperate Dan cow pie (made from one and three-quarter pounds of steak and kidney under an 8-inch-wide pastry crust and decorated with imitation cow horns), and deep-fried Mars Bars and chips. They may be one step ahead of the rest of us, but in essence their high-fat diet only reflects the way our country has been eating for some decades.

Getting Fatter yet Eating Less

Somewhat surprisingly, over the past fifty years we have been steadily decreasing the number of calories we eat per day. The amount of those calories that come from fat, however, has increased. This means that we have been gradually replacing foods such as potatoes, bread and cereals with those rich in oils, margarine, butter and animal blubber. This has several effects.

1. Fats supply twice as many calories as starchy and sugary foods. There are as many calories in the butter or margarine you put on two slices of toast, for example, as in the bread itself.

2. It's easy to overeat fatty foods. Practically everyone knows you can start on a large bar of chocolate and then, quite suddenly, almost without realizing it, find only the wrapper's left. The same goes for crisps, peanuts, cream cakes and fancy biscuits. So are you being a glutton, or does the excuse 'I had no idea I'd eaten all that' hold water? Surprisingly, yes, it does.

   One of those quirks of being human is that the unbelievably complicated mechanisms that get fired off in our brains to tell us we're full don't seem to work very well when it comes to fatty foods. Eat a large piece of chicken bursting with protein and pretty soon your body will be saying, 'Stop – I've had enough.' The same goes for potatoes, rice and bread, if you serve them on their own. The body registers fullness and puts the brakes on eating. With fatty foods, the foods – let's face it – many people eat most of, you can just go on eating. So it's not necessarily just a weak will that conspires against us, it's nature as well.

3. If we are eating more calories than we need on a regular basis, the body has no trouble at all in recognizing the fatty part of the meal or snack and saying, right, off you go to the stomach, bum, hips or wherever your wobbly bits happen to be. It has a great deal of trouble, on the other hand, turning excess sugar, starch and protein into fat.

So what does all this mean? The bottom line is that it's easier to get fat when you eat a lot of fat. The most practical way to cut down on the total amount of fat in your diet is to eat more starchy and sugary foods. If you're thinking, 'Eat more sugary foods? The woman's barking mad. She'll be telling us potatoes aren't fattening next', then you'd be at least part right – potatoes aren't fattening. If you look at populations as a whole you can show time and time again that those who eat more starch and sugar eat less fat, and those who eat more fat eat less starch and sugar.

This phenomenon is called the Sugar–Fat Seesaw. When sugar goes up, fat comes down. When fat goes up, sugar comes down. Since fat has twice the calories of sugar, you can see how eating more sugar can actually help you to lose weight.

How does breakfast help to keep you slim? It's now been demonstrated that the breakfast-skippers among you have higher fat intakes than those who sit down and eat a cereal breakfast before leaving home. This is true for adults, teenagers and children alike. It's also been shown that cereal breakfast-eaters have lower fat intakes than all other people, not just breakfast-skippers. This is probably for several reasons.

First, cereals replace traditional higher-fat foods such as fried toast, eggs, bacon and sausages. Secondly, cereals tip the balance of the day's food intake in the direction of sugar in the sugar–fat seesaw.

Some scientists in Glasgow decided to check out this research to see whether the simple recommendation to eat cereal for breakfast could swing the sugar–fat seesaw and potentially help to stop the relentless march towards a national weight disaster. Sixty normal and slightly overweight women were split into two groups. One group was simply asked to eat 60 grams of breakfast cereal (about two bowls) with semi-skimmed milk, and then to eat as normal for the rest of the day. The other groups was told to eat as normal.

After twelve weeks, sure enough, the amount of fat in the cereal-eaters diets had gone down and the amount of carbohydrate up. The sugar–fat seesaw was moving. Did this have any effect on their weight, even though they weren't trying to lose any? The answer was yes. Those who ate 60 grams of cereal a day effortlessly lost an average of nearly 1.5 kilograms over the twelve weeks. Those women who had been a little overweight at the start of the twelve weeks lost more than that.

Other tests in Glasgow showed that people who were deliberately trying to lose weight managed to shift most when they were advised to follow a low-fat diet but not told to restrict their sugar intakes. After eight weeks those who had tried to limit fat and sugar had lost 2 kilos, whereas those who were told just to restrict fat lost 3 kilos. Another eight weeks later, they had sustained this weight loss. Getting people to concentrate on reducing fat intake seems to be the key to their losing weight. This is just a smallish group of people and the test took place only over a four-month period, but you have to agree it's pretty interesting stuff.

Interesting enough to cause Terry Kirk, who is the senior lecturer in Nutrition at Queen Margaret's College, Glasgow, to say, 'This simple message to increase consumption of breakfast cereals could help achieve targets for weight control and thus improve the health of the nation.' Imagine, a nutritionist saying, yes, go on, eat more of something other than just fruit and vegetables. Sugar-coated cereals, high-fibre cereals, whatever you fancy. Just eat more and you could lose weight. Not bad, eh?

How Else can Breakfast help in the Battle of the Bulge?

As well as altering our sugar–fat seesaw in a fast, convenient and, most importantly, tasty way, eating a cereal breakfast may also help us in other ways to control the amount we eat. For example, it may be that eating the higher-fibre versions can help control our appetite.

When a group of normal-weight women was studied (by Burley in 1997), those fed the high-fibre breakfast seemed to feel fuller over the next three hours than those who weren't, in spite of it being lower in calories than the standard breakfast. Whether this has any real effect in the long term on the amount of food eaten during the rest of the day is unclear, but if you want to keep the mid-morning munchies at bay, one thing is for sure, if you have eaten something for breakfast you're far more likely to succeed.

The importance of appetite control in the battle of the bulge can be seen by looking at the results of a recent NOP survey (Survey for the Breakfast Report, 1997). It showed that 34 per cent of all elevenses-munchers liked to have biscuits, 13 per cent crisps and 12 per cent chocolate. It's easy to see how eating breakfast, and so not eating elevenses, could help keep weight gain at bay.

If eating breakfast stops you nibbling elevenses, it seems likely it will help you to control your weight. The breakdown of regular mealtimes and the move towards 'grazing' and snacking is seen by many obesity experts to be a real problem for those who are prone to gaining weight. As Dr Andrew Prentice, head of the Energy Group at the Medical Research Council Dunn Nutrition Centre in Cambridge, says, 'Breakfast is a key part of the traditional meal pattern. If this first meal of the day breaks down, it doesn't set a very good example for the rest of the day's food intake.'

You don't need to be a qualified nutritionist to know that a rumbling stomach needs filling. Hunger is one of the most powerful feelings we experience. Skipping breakfast means mid-morning munchies are inevitable and are likely to consist of anything you can lay your hands on.

Great Fat Myths of our Time

We know overeating and lack of exercise lead to weight gain, but a surprising number of people will still make excuses. Read these classics. Do they sound familiar?

Being fat is in my genes. My grandma was fat, my mum is fat and I'm fat. Eating breakfast won't make a blind bit of difference

How often have you heard someone say this, and how often have you looked at their family and thought, 'Oh, she's got a point, they're all built like Sumo wrestlers'?

And indeed they would have a point, because obesity and being overweight does appear to run in families. But then you have to ask yourself another question. How active is this family? What kind of a diet do they eat? Is it all down to genetics or is something else playing a role?

It's true that some people are genetically predisposed to be larger than others, but actual body weight has more to do with environmental factors, such as what and how much you eat and how much or little exercise you take, than the genetic pool on which you are drawing.

You may be about to say, 'Yes, but what about Thingymeflip – he eats whatever he likes and doesn't put on a pound.' Does he? How do you know? Are you with him twenty-four hours a day monitoring his food intake? Andrew Prentice and his team up at the Dunn Nutrition Centre *have* monitored people twenty-four hours a day, and they saw just how much truth there was in this old chestnut.

Goodness knows how, but they somehow managed to persuade a group of lean and overweight men to take part in a seven-month experiment in the Dunn Centre's special facility where daily food intake and energy expenditure were accurately measured. During part of the stay they were intentionally overfed by 50 per cent of their required calories. The scientists watched and measured with bated breath. Would the natural skinnies miraculously and spontaneously burn off the excess calories into thin air and thus not gain weight?

No, they didn't. In spite of claiming that they could eat as much as they wished, the lean men put on as much as the fat ones (over 8 kilos in forty-two days). So next time you look enviously at that slim girl tucking into a cream cake, remember – she is compensating for it elsewhere in her diet or is doing loads of exercise to burn it off.

It's my metabolism – I burn fewer calories than slim people, that's why I put on weight

Really? Well, then you must be able to defy the laws of physics. Unless you are one of the minuscule number of people born with a metabolic disease such as Prader Willi syndrome, in which children have insatiable appetites and grow to the most enormous sizes, then the larger you are the higher your metabolic rate. It's a tricky one to grasp, this, and people carrying excess weight will argue until they drop that they are the exception. They are almost certainly not. Studies in the metabolic rooms at the Dunn Centre have shown that the heavier you are, the more calories it takes to keep you alive. And if you stop and think about it, you'll see it must be true. The more there is of you, the more calories are needed to fuel all the cells, and the more calories you need to move your greater weight around. Just as a big Jaguar guzzles far more petrol than a Mini, a 16-stone woman has been shown to burn up around 1,900 calories a day before she has even got out of bed, whereas a 9-stone woman burns up about 1,350.

I don't exercise because I don't want to build up ugly muscles. Anyway, muscles weigh more than fat so I'd only end up heavier

Tosh. Besides eating too much fat, the other major contributor to being overweight during the last fifty years has been the alarming increase in lazy lifestyles. Nowadays only 20 per cent of men and 10 per cent of women are employed in active occupations. The rest of us have adopted almost completely sedentary lifestyles, with energy-saving domestic appliances, motorized transport, mechanized equipment and deskbound jobs turning us into almost complete sloths.

In the Allied Dunbar survey on national fitness carried out in 1992 and the Health Survey for England carried out from 1991, it was revealed that during the four-week period running up to the survey less than 20 per cent of men and women questioned had managed to walk continuously for two miles. Ninety per cent had not cycled and 50–60 per cent had not done any vigorous sport. Only around 25 per cent had done any vigorous activity of any type. The increase in obesity in this country seems to be particularly related to the increase in television viewing and car ownership.

Getting active, whether it's walking, aerobics, the gym, swimming, cycling, squash, tennis, badminton, football, rugby, netball or dancing, helps to build muscle. Muscle burns calories whereas fat stores do not. By increasing muscle you increase your metabolic rate. This will help you burn up fat which, when combined with sensible eating, can help you lose weight, not put it on.

My kids are as skinny as rakes and they hate breakfast. There doesn't seem much point in causing a scene and forcing them to eat it

Habits, whether good or bad, are hard to break. If you lay down the foundations of good habits now, your children are more likely to continue with them into adulthood. They may not be overweight now, but who knows what lies ahead of them? If they aren't eating breakfast you can be sure they'll be tucking into something pretty soon after they've left home, and that something will probably take the form of a high-fat snack. Why not give them the chance to start the way you'd like them to go on? Do all you can to get them to have breakfast before leaving home. It takes five minutes to eat and the effects could last a lifetime.

Chapter 9

How Breakfast may help beat Breast Cancer

How, you may well ask, can eating breakfast help in the fight against breast cancer? In several ways. For one, by helping to control body weight. There's a whole chapter on how breakfast is able to do this (Chapter 8), which is worth checking out. In a nutshell, in tests, people who skipped breakfast have been found to weigh more than those who sat down for something to eat before leaving home.

This relates to breast cancer because it has been shown that women who gain weight during their adult life are more prone to developing breast cancer than those who maintain a sensible, stable weight. Precisely why gaining weight has this effect is not clear, but it may be because fat cells secrete a substance that contains a hormone called aromatase. Aromatase seems to be able to convert normally circulating male hormones (which all women have in small amounts, just as all men have some female hormones) into female ones. These extra female hormones may then stimulate cell division in breast tissue which could in some women become cancerous.

Next comes the observation that women who have diets that are rich in wholegrain cereals have lower rates of breast cancer. The reason for this is again down to levels of circulating female hormones. There is a lot of indirect evidence to suggest that women with diets that are low in wholegrain cereals have higher levels of oestrogens in their blood and are more at risk of breast cancer than those who have less. This seems to be again because increased amounts of female hormones, particularly oestrogen, stimulate cell division in the breast, cells which may spin out of control and turn cancerous.

70

The Wholegrain Story

Women who live in countries where the incidence of breast cancer is low, for example China, have on average 36 per cent lower oestrogen levels than women in Britain. Japanese women also have lower levels. The strange thing is, if they move to Western societies, rates of breast cancer increase within a generation.

Diets and lifestyles differ widely between Asian and Western countries, but the observations are none the less interesting. If you compare the oestrogen levels of vegetarian women in the West and of those who eat a mixed diet, the same trend shows up. Vegetarians, who eat more wholegrain foods, have lower levels of oestrogen.

Thinking there could be a link, researchers started doing tests to see what it is about diets high in wholegrain cereals that reduces oestrogen levels. They pretty soon saw that it has something to do with the bowel. This link may seem odd. What on earth have levels of oestrogen in the blood got to do with what's in the bowel? Quite a lot, it turns out.

Oestrogens don't just stay in the blood. They undergo a complicated circuit around several organs. The journey begins in the ovaries where they are produced. They then go into the blood and happily circulate until it's time for them to be taken to the liver, where they are either prepared to be lost from the body in the urine, or are sent via the gall bladder and bile duct to the bowel to be lost in the stool.

However, some of the oestrogens that are sent to the bowel can be reabsorbed from the stools into the bloodstream, which pushes up total circulating levels of oestrogen. This is where diets rich in wholegrain cereals come in. They speed up the passage of the stools through the gut. This is a bit like the oestrogens being on an Intercity 125. They can't get off because the train is going too fast. Trapped as they are in the faster-moving stool, they leave the body instead of being reabsorbed. This seems to have the effect of lowering total blood oestrogen levels.

Studies have now been done on how wholegrain wheat fibre has this effect. There's a very large study taking place at the moment, which will eventually reveal whether lowering oestrogen levels reduces the number of women who develop breast cancer. Meanwhile, the hunch is pretty strong that it will, so why not up your wholewheat consumption anyway? It certainly won't do you any harm, and may protect you not just from breast cancer but also from bowel cancer. Breakfast is the easiest meal at which to take this positive health step by regularly including cereals such as All-Bran Plus, All-Bran Bite Size, Optima Fruit 'n' Fibre, Healthwise Bran Flakes, Frosted Wheats, Weetabix and Shredded Wheat, along with 100 per cent wholemeal bread.

Plant Oestrogens

Diets rich in wholegrain cereals may have one more protective effect. This time it comes in the form of substances known as isoflavones and lignans, found in foods like wholemeal bread and wholegrain breakfast cereals. These substances are known as plant oestrogens.

Oestrogens that circulate in the blood seem to be able to latch on to cells in the breast. Once they have latched on they appear to switch on a process that makes the cells divide and multiply. They act like a key in a lock. It is possible that plant oestrogens are able to fit on to the same 'locks' as human oestrogens, but the key doesn't really fit, so they are not able to switch on the same cell division. By filling up the locks yet not causing any effect, the theory is they are able to reduce the negative effects of human oestrogens. Taking a look around the world, at countries where lots of plant oestrogens are eaten on a daily basis, rates of breast cancer are again lower.

The take-home message from all of this is to increase your daily intake of wholegrain wheat. Breakfast is one of the easiest and most palatable meals at which to do this.

Chapter 10

Breakfast and Colon Cancer

A recent survey carried out by the Cancer Research Campaign showed that a quarter of all adults knew someone who had been diagnosed with, or treated for, bowel cancer. Someone probably very like Cathy Richards.

Cathy was just thirty-six back in 1976 when she found out she had bowel cancer. After a successful operation she fully recovered, and has now not only seen her children grow up but is keeping a watchful eye over her growing clutch of grandchildren. Here's her story.

'I was a young, active and happy mum of four great children aged two to fifteen. I had a healthy lifestyle living in Pembrokeshire. Then, all of a sudden, in 1976 I started to feel unwell. I was totally washed out and listless for apparently no reason at all. I had had trouble with piles around five to six months previously but the doctor kept treating them and sending me home. Other than that, I'd been anaemic when my youngest son was eleven months and at the time had suffered with some bleeding rectally. I was told then that it wouldn't be wise to go into hospital to have it checked since I was still breastfeeding, so I forgot all about it. Looking back, that was probably the start of my trouble.

'It was the tiredness which made me go back to my doctor and insist that I saw someone else for a second opinion. That Friday I saw a general physician who checked my bowel with the help of a microscopic camera. He said I had a bad ulcer and needed to come straight into hospital on the Monday. I said, By ulcer, do you mean cancer? and he said, Yes, probably.

'Sure enough the next Tuesday I had a young doctor standing at my bed asking me where I wanted the colostomy bag sited, which I would need after the operation on my cancer.

It was bizarre. They took away the cancer which it turned out was at the very lowest end of the bowel. These days they can do the operation and you won't need a permanent bag. I've had mine for twenty-two years and it's not really a problem. It was not having help to deal with the diagnosis that worried me. These days you can pick up a phone and talk to people; those days it was different.

'Having said that, people are still so worried about talking about their bowels. We are so Victorian about it. You will hear people openly discuss sex, Aids and breast cancer, but not mention anything about down there. It's so short-sighted. I would beg people to keep an eye on things. If you notice any changes at all in how often you go to the loo, any sudden constipation or diarrhoea, any weight loss, tiredness, or general discomfort when you go, then check it out with your GP. They are very geared up now and there's no need to die from it if you catch it early. Poor Bobby Moore was a prime case. He didn't get help soon enough. It doesn't need to be like that.'

It's no good frightening you with statistics – that's rarely effective – but when it comes to bowel cancer it's difficult not to mention some basic facts. Were you aware, for example, that some forty-nine people die every day in the UK from this disease, a good half of whom could have been saved by some simple dietary changes? Staggering, isn't it?

Of course hereditary factors play a role in the development of bowel cancer, accounting for around one out of ten cases. It also has to be appreciated that bowel cancer is caused by a complex combination of factors, not just a lousy diet. But the fact remains that if your doctor told you that you could dramatically reduce yours and your family's risk of this country's number-two cancer killer just by eating more wholegrain cereals, vegetables and fruits, you'd probably want to hear more.

How can Cereals and Vegetables fight Colon Cancer?

Long before Audrey Eyton's F-Plan Diet introduced the nation to the word 'fibre', scientists thought that there could be a link between diets rich in wholegrain cereals, vegetables and fruits, and protection against diseases of the bowel, including both the large intestine (or colon) and the rectum. Have a look at the diagram.

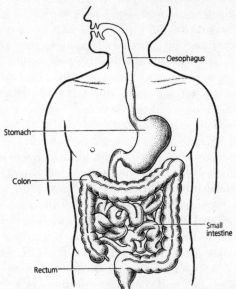

The bowel is made up of the colon, approximately 3 feet (1 metre) in length, and the rectum ,which is just 6 inches (16cm).

Even as far back as 400BC, the great physician Hippocrates was recommending the eating of wholemeal bread for its 'salutary effects upon the bowels'. Yet somewhere in the last 200 years we lost touch with whole foods and found, unlike all other plant-eating animals, ways to refine our food.

One of the most famous people in the world of colon health and disease was a distinguished doctor called Dennis Burkitt. Now his interest in analysing stools isn't everyone's cup of tea. But thank goodness he took the trouble to do this, both in the UK and in many parts of Africa. For it was through looking at the consistency and weight of stool that he came up with his theory on how eating plant foods in the form nature intended, that is unrefined with all their tough cell walls intact, could help prevent many diseases associated with the bowel.

His theory was that a fair part of these foods was left undigested by the upper intestine and passed on into the bowel. Here, he believed, this material was fermented by the millions and millions of bacteria which call the bowel their home. This fermentation process, he claimed, substantially increased the weight of the stool. This in turn had the effect of diluting any potential cancer-causing substances lurking in the bowel. Along with the dilution of these toxins came the advantage that, because the stools weighed more, the speed at which they passed out of the body increased. This gave the carcinogens still less chance to wreak havoc and set up cancerous sites on the bowel walls.

Burkitt and his colleagues documented the weight of waste matter and the length of time it took to pass through. Passage time was measured from the moment a food is eaten until its waste material was passed in the stools. They found that there were large differences between Ugandan villagers, who ate lots of whole foods, and UK inhabitants, who ate a great deal fewer. The average Ugandan villager produced 470 grams of stool a day, which took thirty-six hours to pass. The UK figures were alarmingly different. The average Briton produced just 104 grams of stool per day and took over eighty-three hours to pass them. British vegetarians fared better, with 225 grams of stool which passed through in forty-two hours.

These observations emerged in the 1970s and are largely thought still to be true today, although now some extra ideas have been thrown into the melting pot involving the complicated effects of high-carbohydrate diets on the pH of the bowel. They make the bowel more acidic, and this is thought to reduce the activity of toxins by helping to prevent their build-up.

The rates of colon cancer around the world bear out the theory that wholegrain diets and diets rich in vegetables and fruits reduce bowel cancer. In developing countries where diets are still wholesome and often unrefined, the rates of colon cancer are lower than in developed countries, where we rely on refined versions of flour, bread, rice and pasta, and where our intakes of vegetables and fruits are on the low side. When people from Africa and Asia, where rates of bowel cancer are low, move to high-risk westernized countries, their risk of developing bowel cancer increases, which adds further weight to the whole idea. Clearly a strong environmental factor plays a role in bowel cancer, a factor which is commonly agreed to be diet.

While parts of our population are happy to chomp away on 100 per cent raw foods (fruitarians and very strict vegans, to mention a couple), most of us would, in reality, find it hard to turn back the clock and pretend we'd never tasted the delights produced by the modern food industry. So it's fortunate that modern food science has made it possible to create attractive and appetizing wholegrain options, which as well as tickling our fancy, will do us good on the inside too.

Some wholesome Foods

Wholegrain breakfast cereals such as All-Bran Plus, All-Bran Bite Size, Fruit 'n' Fibre, Bran Flakes, Oat Flakes, Weetabix, Fibre 1 and Shredded Wheat, and 100 per cent wholemeal bread, muffins, fruit scones and pitta are all ways of improving the wholegrain fibre at breakfast time.

Added Bonus

The role that wholegrain cereals, especially wheat, plus fruits and vegetables play in preventing bowel cancer may not end with their ability to bulk out the stools and increase the number of times we need to go to the loo. They may also help by supplying us with vital antioxidants and other substances that have anti-carcinogenic effects in the bowel.

Phytate, for example, which is found in the large intestine as a result of eating wholegrain cereals, can bind potentially carcinogenic materials and render them harmless. So too can flavonols and tannins found in the undigested parts of vegetables. One last advantage of a diet rich in wholegrain cereals, fruits and vegetables is highlighted by another famous

UK bowel specialist, Dr Kenneth Heaton, who once wrote that such diets 'will be rich in micronutrients and potassium and low in fat, sugar and sodium. Such a diet combines virtually all the internationally accepted guidelines to healthy eating.'

How to Eat to Beat Bowel Cancer

Breakfast is one of the easiest meals at which to pack in unrefined cereals. Since wheat is the cereal that seems to have the most protective effect, why not go for the following combinations:

For unrefined wheat choose a bowl of All-Bran Plus, All-Bran Bite Size, Fruit 'n' Fibre, Bran Flakes, Sultana Bran, Weetabix, Shredded Wheat or Fibre 1 with skimmed or semi-skimmed milk. Add one or two slices of wholemeal bread or toast, rye bread or wholemeal muffins.

For fruit or vegetables try a chopped-up banana, a grated apple or a glass of fruit or vegetable juice.

If you get **mid-morning munchies**, be prepared. Have something like a wholemeal fruit scone or a piece of fruit at hand to quell the hunger.

Lunch depends very much on the type of life you lead. Whether you are based at home, in an office or are continually on the run, it's wise to make time for something to eat to keep you going in the afternoon ahead. If it's a quick sandwich go for wholemeal bread or pitta bread. If you like pasta or rice salads choose those made with brown pasta or wholegrain brown rice. If you have to go out for lunch, try the trusted baked potato with a filling of beans and a salad to go with it. If there's nothing wholesome and wholegrain on the menu, make sure you at least get some vegetables and, if possible, fruit as well.

Who doesn't get **4.00 p.m. cravings**? Fill the gap until suppertime with anything from ready-to-eat dried fruit that you can eat at your desk or on the move, to wholegrain crispbreads with a little cheese, some fresh fruit or another bowl of wholegrain breakfast cereal. What better low-fat snack to plug the hunger?

For **dinner** start buying in the wholegrain versions of pasta and rice. If you and your family don't fancy going the whole hog, begin by going half and half. It's amazing how quickly you get the taste for the wholegrain versions and how incredibly filling they seem compared to the refined versions. If you're serving bread with the meal, try to make it wholemeal, and add another vegetable to the dish whenever you get the chance.

Did You Know?

- In rural Africa, where they eat a lot more unrefined foods than people do in the West, the average time taken for foods to pass through the digestive system is thirty-six hours. In the UK it is three days, and sometimes, in the elderly, up to two weeks.
- Breakfast is the easiest meal of the day at which to pack in unrefined wheat. Recent research showed that individuals who regularly took an unrefined cereal for breakfast were the only people to get close to the recommended level of intake. Just one bowl of All-Bran Plus or Fibre 1 supplies a massive half of the daily amount we should be aiming for.
- Piles are in part caused by straining to go to the loo. Increasing unrefined cereals plus fruit and vegetables in the diet takes away the strain and helps keep piles in their place.
- Of all the people questioned in a recent survey by the Cancer Research Campaign and Kellogg's, some 41 per cent were surprised to learn that half of all bowel cancer cases could be prevented by eating a diet high in cereal fibre.
- The same survey showed that only 31 per cent of 15–20-year-olds eats a diet containing plenty of cereals, fruit and vegetables.

- Bowel cancer may only start to show up once you hit your forties but you are building up your risk throughout life. Changing your diet whatever your age will add to your protection.
- Sixty-two per cent of all patients who went to their GP had no idea that their bowel symptoms were down to bowel cancer.
- The message from this chapter is that increasing your intake of wholegrain cereals, fruits and vegetables seems to help reduce yours and your family's risk of developing bowel cancer. Start increasing intakes now.

Chapter 11

Strong Bones for Life

What do you think of when you hear the word 'osteoporosis'? That it's a problem that affects old ladies? That it's got something to do with weak bones? Well, you'd be correct on both fronts, but that's only part of the story.

For example, did you know that thanks to osteoporosis (which literally means thinning of the bones), every three minutes in this country someone sustains a fracture? That one in three women is affected but one in twelve men is too? Or that £750 million of the health budget is spent on mending hip fractures, and that within just six months of sustaining the injury, some 20 per cent of those affected will die. That's 15,000 women a year dying from osteoporosis. So you see it's not just a bit of a problem that old people have to live with, people can die from it too.

That's the bad news. The good news is that osteoporosis is both treatable and preventable. We may have the image that bones are solid masses that remain the same throughout our entire life. Nothing could be further from the truth. Bones are made up of a network of protein tissue, which comprises one third of their weight. Onto this protein network, crystalline minerals such as calcium are constantly being deposited and removed. The minerals make up the other two-thirds of a bone's weight. Bones are just as alive as the rest of our bodies, and every year a good 10 per cent of your skeleton has been remodelled.

Calcium for Life

During the years of rapid growth children's and teenagers' bones lengthen and harden. This stops around the age of nineteen, when the bones make up about a sixth of total body weight. From birth, when we have just 30 grams of calcium in our body, to fully grown adulthood, the bones need to accumulate some 1,170 grams of calcium from the diet. This requires a daily intake of around 550 milligrams up to the age of ten, about 1,000 milligrams a day from eleven to eighteen and around 800 milligrams a day from there on. Calcium is needed every day in childhood to help bones grow, and in adulthood to maintain them in good condition.

In teenagers a shortage of calcium will stunt growth so that full height potential is not reached. This is only the start of the problems. Not only will full height not be reached, the bones which do develop may not reach what's known as their 'peak bone density'. In other words, they won't have as much calcium on the protein superstructure as they could or should have.

This immediately puts a person at a disadvantage because later in life the bones naturally start to lose some of this density. This is particularly so for women once they have reached the menopause. Bone density is at its maximum until our early thirties, and from then on it's all downhill. Not that the loss is particularly rapid to start with. Initially we lose about 1 per cent a year. Once women reach the menopause, this increases to a 2–3 per cent loss annually. This means that by the age of seventy, around one third of bone mass could be lost. Obviously the higher your bone density is to start with, the more you will have left as these natural processes occur.

The mineral content of a woman's bones at the time of menopause is much more a result of her calcium intakes over the previous four or five decades than over the last few years, so it's vital to ensure that good calcium habits are ingrained from the youngest age possible.

Iris Swain is a 73-year-old from Wolverhampton who suffers from osteoporosis. She believes that getting this message across to young girls is vital. 'I'm an ex-deputy head of a seventeen-hundred-pupil secondary school. Young people of today don't understand what they are setting in store for tomorrow. They have no idea that osteoporosis means that your bones become like Crunchy Bars. Imagine sinking your teeth into a Crunchy Bar. It sort of loses its shape. That's what happens to your bones. Bones become spongy. In your spine this means they collapse, which makes it curve and shrink. You become bent over, which in turn dislodges your internal organs through the extra pressure, so your whole body is affected. When I see girls trying to be as skinny as those models on the catwalks it worries me. They are very likely to have problems with their bones in the future. We have to encourage them not to smoke, to take regular weight-bearing exercise and of course to take more calcium. I can't take enough milk. I have it in and on my porridge for breakfast, in sauces, custard and even blanc-manges. I can't get on with yoghurts but I do eat plenty of calcium-rich cheese and greens as well.'

Dairy products, especially milk, are one of the very best sources of calcium. It is not just that milk is an incredibly rich source, it's also that the calcium in milk seems to be absorbed better by the body than the calcium in other foods. If you look at the table below you can see the number of servings of other calcium-containing foods you need to eat to get the same amount of calcium in a 240 ml glass of milk.

Food	Typical serving size	Number of servings needed
Milk	240 ml glass	1
Almonds, dry roasted	28 grams	5.7
Beans, red kidney	172 grams	14
Broccoli	71 grams	5.2
Cabbage	75 grams	5.9
Cauliflower	62 grams	8.2
Sesame seeds	28 grams	12.5
Spinach	90 grams	15.5
Sprouts	78 grams	8
Watercress	17 grams	7.2

A pint of milk, whether it's skimmed, semi-skimmed or whole, supplies at least 670 milligrams of calcium – that's almost all of your day's requirement. Although it's relatively simple to reach 700 milligrams a day by consuming milk and dairy products like yoghurt and cheese, a government survey showed that as many as one in four teenage girls aged fourteen to fifteen and young women aged sixteen to eighteen have inadequate calcium intakes (eleven- to eighteen-year-old girls are judged in the UK to need 800 milligrams a day). If you were to measure their intakes against American recommendations of 1,200 milligrams a day, then an even larger number of girls would be woefully down on their calcium.

Figures for intakes in all age groups are higher in the United States. Recent studies on teenagers based on their bone density led a group of American scientists to go one step further and suggest upping intakes to 1,200–1,500 milligrams during growth, with 1,000 milligrams for women up to fifty. From fifty on they say those not on hormone replacement therapy need 1,500 milligrams a day, while those on HRT can stick to 1,000 milligrams. All men and women over sixty-five should, in their opinion, be getting 1,500 milligrams a day.

How to get enough Calcium

Food	Serving	Calcium content
Milk	190 ml	230 mg
All-Bran Plus	40 grams	114 mg
Baked beans	110 grams	50 mg
Broccoli	110 grams	85 mg
Cheddar cheese	28 grams	205 mg
Cottage cheese	80 grams	60 mg
Dried apricots	56 grams	52 mg
Ice cream	2 scoops	134 mg
Orange	1 large	58 mg
Sardines with bones	56 grams	220 mg
Shelled prawns	84 grams	126 mg
Yoghurt	150 ml (small carton)	240 mg

Clearly dairy products are the richest source of calcium in the diet. These days you can get milks and yoghurts with added calcium from many supermarkets, and some soya milks are enriched with calcium as well. Evidence that intake of dairy foods improves bone density has been shown by comparing diet and bone mass in groups of people. It has also been shown by testing calcium intakes in identical twins. Seventy pairs of identical twins aged six to fourteen were used in one study. One of each pair was given 1,612 milligrams of calcium a day and the other 908 milligrams. The children who had the higher intakes had greater density of bone over the three years they were studied than those on the lower intakes. The amount of increase in density could over an extended period of time have resulted in a 30–40 per cent reduction in fractures.

Calcium in the form of milk has been shown to improve deposits on the bone by up to 10 per cent. Given this, encouraging youngsters to consume more milk can only be a good thing. Breakfast is one of the easiest meals at which to get milk into kids, and ourselves, primarily through pouring it over breakfast cereals, hot or cold. In an average bowl you would use at least 125 millilitres. In addition you could try adding yoghurt to cereal, or use milk and yoghurt plus some fruit to create a shake. Adding chopped almonds, sunflower seeds, dried figs and dried apricots would also improve intakes. Encouraging the use of cereal and milk as snacks at other times of the day means you can increase intakes further still.

Calcium needs Vitamin D

It's all very well getting lots of calcium from the foods you eat and drink, but there's another part to the jigsaw. Calcium needs vitamin D for it to be absorbed into the body and deposited on the bone. In this country most of us should in theory from the age of four right through to sixty-five be getting enough vitamin D without worrying about how much we eat in foods (pregnant women need 10 micrograms a day from food). This is because vitamin D is formed under the skin when sunlight shines on it, which means roughly from the end of March through to the end of October. During the winter we survive on the vitamin D stores we have built up during the summer.

However, not all of us build up sufficient vitamin D, especially if we don't get out much during the summer days or don't expose, say, our arms and legs to the sunlight. It has been discovered that women between forty-five and sixty-five might be able to increase their bone density by 5–10 per cent if vitamin D levels in the blood were raised, and that elderly people can reduce fracture rates in as little as eighteen months when treated with vitamin D.

Although dietary sources of this vitamin are limited – for example it is found in oily fish, eggs, butter and whole milk – it is added to many breakfast cereals, which provides the added bonus for having a cereal and milk start to the day. A bowl of Special K, for example, served with semi-skimmed milk, supplies 2.5 micrograms of vitamin D.

What do you get from your Cereal's Milk?

Type of milk	Calories	Fat	Protein	Calcium
Whole	83	5 grams	4 grams	144 mg
Semi-skimmed	58	2 grams	4 grams	150 mg
Skimmed	41	0.1 grams	4 grams	150 mg

Living with Osteoporosis

Iris Swain continues: 'I became aware of osteoporosis because it was in my family. I fell over eight years ago and fractured my wrist. It was one of those silly situations. My brother was being ordained and I was rushing to whip the clingfilm off the sandwiches for the buffet afterwards. I just slipped and that was that. It should have rung bells with the physios and doctors because wrist fractures are the first sign of osteoporosis but it was me who made the link. I insisted on having a bone scan and sure enough my bone density was low. I am losing height and my mobility isn't what it was. I can still get around but I won't go out if it snows or is icy. You are affected in many ways. For example, I've had problems with my teeth: you don't think of that, do you? I'm not as badly affected as many people. Some people's quality of life is virtually non-existent. They can become totally dependent on others, and eventually die from the bone weakness. We need to get this message across.'

Mrs Joan Farnham, 60, from Sussex, says: 'I've always been incredibly fit physically and am the first on the dancefloor given half a chance. I was at a barn dance with some friends while on holiday in Cyprus. I was bombing around with my husband when suddenly his foot tripped on an uneven piece of flooring. We both fell heavily and I landed on my left hip, which got badly fractured. Getting back to England took days and days to organize and when I eventually arrived home I had a hip replacement. The first one didn't work so nine months later I had a second one. The bone in my hip was very poor. I started taking regular exercise and supplements and sorted out my diet. I'm glad to say the density of the hip has increased since two years ago. Once you've had this kind of shock you start to take things seriously. If only we could get young people to do this early on.'

Malcolm Stewart, 43, from Chesterfield, says: 'I've always had very bad asthma and have been on steroids for years. For a good two years solidly I couldn't do without them. They control my asthma but a side-effect is that my bones lost density and my spine collapsed. I can't work now because I can't guarantee to be able to do more than two or three days in a row. Mine is an extreme example caused by drugs but what I'd like to get across is that men need to think about their bone health too. Men seem to have less information about health and how to look after themselves than women, but they really need to take note. I thought osteoporosis was a problem only post-menopausal women had, but it affects men as well. I grew up in a time when we did lots of exercise, had school milk and a decent school dinner. Things have changed these days. I keep an eye on my boys, making sure they don't go out without breakfast because that's one meal I can make sure they are getting milk in. We need to think about the boys and their lifestyles and diets as well as the young girls.'

Chapter 12

Boost your Iron at Breakfast

Iron is a vital nutrient, found in the highest amounts in red meat. It is also in some nuts and dried fruits, and breakfast cereals that have had it added. It's essential because the body uses it to make haemoglobin, the substance in blood that not only gives it its bright red colour but also carries oxygen around to all the cells and organs that keep us alive. Haemoglobin is a bit like a freight train, picking oxygen up from the lungs and dropping it off where it's needed most. If we don't eat enough iron then haemoglobin levels fall and less oxygen is able to be carried around. This eventually leads to iron-deficiency anaemia, two of the main symptoms of which are tiredness and a lack of concentration. Although these are the things we may notice most, too little iron also increases the threshold at which you feel pain, interferes with your body's temperature-control systems, decreases your working capacity and leaves the immune system under the weather. As you can imagine, any of these symptoms can seriously affect your enjoyment of everyday life.

Worldwide, anaemia is a serious problem. It is estimated that half the children in Africa and South Asia are anaemic. Some quarter of a billion children are affected in developing countries, which leads to, among many other things, lower IQs, which hamper them further in their struggle for survival.

It's not just developing countries that are affected. In Britain women and teenage girls are particularly at risk of low iron intakes. This is partly down to not eating enough and partly down to some women losing more than average amounts of iron through menstruation. In this country most women get around 12.3 milligrams of iron a day, when the recommended amount is more like 15 milligrams. For those who have heavy menstrual losses around 17 milligrams is recommended. Older people who perhaps don't have very good diets and whose ability to absorb iron from foods decreases with age may also be prone to deficiencies and therefore anaemia.

Addressing the Problem

Dr Mike Nelson, a nutritionist at King's College at London University, believes that between 10 and 20 per cent of apparently healthy girls could have low iron levels, which affects their ability to concentrate in school and thus their ability to learn. 'Girls who are dieting and those switching to a vegetarian diet are particularly at risk,' he explains. 'New vegetarians are most at risk in the first year of conversion often because they cut out meat and don't know how to replace the iron from the meat with other foods. Girls who diet and go vegetarian at the same time are particularly at risk and may like to think about eating fortified foods or even taking a modest supplement.'

Increasing iron intakes could make all the difference with school work. Nelson concludes: 'In tests we have carried out we think that the difference in IQ between girls who get enough iron in their diets and those who are anaemic can mean the difference between a D and C grade in GCSEs.'

But it's not just teenage girls who should take note. It has also been shown that at least 12 per cent of women who visit antenatal clinics have low iron levels. Since they are offered iron supplements, the problem can at least be addressed. Perhaps more worrying are the numbers of people who are going about their daily lives far less effectively and efficiently than they could be, thanks to a simple shortage of the mineral iron.

Nelson says: 'We get only about 3 per cent of our iron from meat but it is very well absorbed. More like 40 to 50 per cent comes from cereal products such as bread and fortified cereals. It's been estimated that an average 30-gram bowl of fortified cereal, for example, supplies 20 per cent of the day's iron needs for kids. That's a good couple of milligrams.'

Sources of Iron in the Diet

The table that follows shows how much iron is in some of the foods we eat.

Food	Quantity of Iron
Kellogg's Sultana Bran, 50-gram Portion-Pak	9 milligrams
Kellogg's All-Bran Plus, 60-gram Portion-Pak	9 milligrams
Kellogg's Healthwise Bran Flakes, 30 grams	7 milligrams
Kellogg's Special K, 30 grams	7 milligrams
Beef, 150 grams	6 milligrams
Baked beans, 200 grams	5 milligrams
Dhal, 155 grams	5 milligrams
Spinach, 130 grams	5 milligrams
Kellogg's Optima Fruit 'n' Fibre, 50-gram Portion-Pak	4 milligrams
Sardines, tinned, 85 grams	4 milligrams
Eggs, 2 boiled	3 milligrams
Figs, 4	3 milligrams
Leeks, boiled, 125 grams	3 milligrams
Pilchards, tinned, 105 grams	3 milligrams
Weetabix, 50 grams	3 milligrams
Cashew nuts, 40 grams	2 milligrams
Muesli, 50 grams	2 milligrams
Raspberries, 15	2 milligrams
Wholemeal bread, 2 slices	2 milligrams
Shreddies, 50 grams	1 milligram

Absorbing the Iron we Eat

Knowing how much iron is in foods is one side of the story. The other is to know which foods and drinks increase the absorption of iron, and which decrease it. Take a look at the list below and then look at the types of breakfast which not only supply good amounts of iron but also offer the best chance of absorption.

Substances that decrease Iron Absorption

Tannin – found in tea
Egg proteins
Phytates – found in foods such as spinach

Substances that improve Iron Absorption

Vitamin C – found in citrus fruits such as oranges, fruit juices such as orange and grapefruit juice, kiwi fruits, red, green and yellow peppers, dark green leafy vegetables
 Fruit sugars – found in fruit juices and all fruits

Good Iron-boosting Breakfast Combinations

Bowl of fortified cereal
Glass of orange juice
Two slices of wholemeal toast with marmalade, honey or
 Marmite

Bowl of fortified cereal with chopped kiwi fruit
Hot croissant with jam
Glass of sparkling water

Yoghurt and figs topped with crushed Bran Flakes
Glass of grapefruit juice

Apple and Date All-Bran with fromage frais
Glass of carrot and apple juice

To Supplement or not to Supplement

If your GP advises you to take iron supplements, then that is the best course of action. If you are taking them yourself as a tonic, stick to supplements that supply 15 milligrams a day. Although tests show that you'd have to have 100 grams of iron a day before it became toxic, what's the point in taking more than you need? Iron supplements can cause constipation, so if you can get your requirements through food, that may be preferable.

Chapter 13

Lifestages

As you will have seen in previous chapters, there are plenty of good reasons for sitting down (or standing up for that matter) to have the first meal of the day. Does our age in any way affect what we should be eating for breakfast? Are some choices more important for certain people than others? Are there any times in our lives when we should be thinking about which nutrients our breakfast is providing? The answer to all these questions is yes.

Infants

Get infants into good habits from the word go by making sure breakfast is on the menu. Weaning from the breast or bottle usually takes place around four to six months of age. By this time the infant's own stores of iron are running low and the mineral needs to be provided by foods. Special infant cereals often have added vitamins and minerals: choose the right one for your child's age. You can make them up with formula milks. The milk designed for children of six months-plus, known as 'follow on' milk, usually has added iron as well.

Mashed banana, puréed pear or apple with yoghurt and scrambled eggs thoroughly cooked also make good breakfasts. Never give your infant skimmed milk. It doesn't contain enough calories, vitamin A or essential fats. Also, don't try weaning them straight on to the F-Plan Diet. There is a right time for introducing high-fibre foods and this isn't it. During this period of rapid development they need energy-dense foods to help them achieve maximum growth. Too many fibre-rich foods will make them feel full and stop them eating before they have consumed enough nutrients.

Karen Knight, a mother of three from West Sussex, remembers the weaning days: 'At least with little ones they are always hungry in the morning so there's none of this not wanting breakfast business. I started all of mine on baby rice and to stop any problems with constipation added a little stewed apple. They all adored the orange-flavoured rice (which I didn't mind finishing, it was very good!). Then I moved them on to baby porridge. Initially I just mixed it in with the rice then gradually added more porridge. By the time they were one they had discovered sugar-coated cereals which they'd have every day if I let them. I liked them to have some variety so I'd buy various cereals and make them try different ones so that they got used to different tastes and textures.'

Toddlers

Although they are not growing at such an incredibly fast rate as infants do, one- to five-year-old children are more prone than infants to nutritional deficiencies because they have used up stores of nutrients built up while in the womb. And being very young, they haven't a chance to accumulate the reserves found in adults. It's also important to remember that little people have little stomachs that get full quickly. The food they are eating needs to be packed with as many nutrients as possible. Foods which supply 'empty calories', in other words calories but no vitamins and minerals, such as sweets, should be kept to a minimum or given only once a proper meal has been eaten. Very few toddlers will refuse breakfast if offered it. Their appetites are still controlled naturally and waking up signals the need to eat before starting the day ahead.

Toddlers need plenty of calcium and vitamin D to help them build their growing bones, and vitamin A to improve their resistance to disease. Starting the day with a fortified cereal containing vitamins D and A, and whole or semi-skimmed milk (only use semi-skimmed after the age of two, and only if your child is growing properly) for calcium and protein, is ideal. A well-cooked boiled or poached egg served with bread and butter is an alternative start: the egg and butter contain vitamins A and D and the bread some calcium. Smooth peanut butter on toast is another option, served with a glass of fruit juice.

Don't forget. This is not the age to be applying strict low-fat rules. Children need fat in their diet not only to provide fat-soluble vitamins A, D and E but also to give them the essential fats that help their nervous system and all their new cells develop properly. Last but not least, it helps to ensure they get enough energy.

Like infants, one- to five-year-olds also need plenty of iron so that as they grow their blood stays healthy and strong. Fortified breakfast cereals are an excellent way of supplying iron at the first meal of the day.

Five- to eleven-year-olds

Surveys show that at this age children are still keen to eat breakfast if you make the time for them to do so. The vast majority are still relying on their finely tuned body-clocks to tell them when it's time to eat. Although at this age they are able to express and assert their own likes and dislikes, this is no time to be giving into any child's whimsical notions that breakfast doesn't count. It does. Studies have shown, as we have seen, that children who go to school on a good breakfast perform better than those who go to classes on an empty stomach.

Always make time for breakfast. A modern breakfast takes no more than ten minutes from start to finish. A packet of cereal takes no time to pour out, cover with milk and eat. Toast takes no longer to prepare. Topped with peanut butter and accompanied by a glass of cool milk and a quick slug of orange juice, this also is a quick and nutritious way to start the day for a change. Just getting the kids to carry out this simple morning ritual will mean their average intake of many nutrients is above those of their friends who rush from the house skipping the first meal of the day. If your kids say they're not hungry, make sure they are not eating too late at night and that they are not going to sleep too late.

Teeth can benefit from breakfast too. Kids of this age are most susceptible to tooth decay if they expose their newly erupting permanent teeth to sugar between meals in the form of sweets and drinks. Giving them breakfast means they are less likely to snack on such foods between meals. If you're worried about the sugar content in sugar-coated cereals then it's important to get the issue into perspective. An average bowl of pre-sweetened cereal contains about 12 grams of sugar: that's about the same amount of sugar you get in a medium-sized apple.

As long as they are growing properly you can start introducing fully skimmed milk to this age group, though they will still be fine on semi-skimmed if they prefer the taste. Both types contain as much (actually a little more) calcium as whole milk, so they will be getting this essential mineral for their growing bones. There's still no need to go completely overboard with wholemeal everything. You can start introducing more fibrous ranges of cereal and wholemeal bread if they like them, but don't get wound up if they like sugar-coated cereals, ask for sugar on the more fibrous ones and have to have marmalade to make the wholemeal bread go down. The amount of sugar these breakfasts contain doesn't add significantly to the total day's intake and brushing their teeth afterwards helps prevent any potential decay problem.

At weekends, when there's more time, you could try serving a cooked breakfast. If you like the full monty on Sundays then try our Grill-up suggestion on page 121, or try the kids out on grilled kippers: they supply loads of vitamin D, which helps calcium absorption, and stacks of the essential fats needed for their developing brains.

Breakfast is a good time to get in some of the day's fruit: either in fruit juices, or by chopping or grating fruit onto cereals, or by blending them with milk to make a fruit shake.

Teenagers

No one needs telling that this is a time when the body makes great spurts in growth. Keeping up with the calcium requirements can be tough for both sexes as they try to accumulate the 1 kilogram-plus of this mineral needed for a strong adult skeleton. Older girls in the UK have been found to be getting less calcium than is recommended. In the fifteen age-group, girls are consuming around 60 per cent less than the government suggested intake of 800 milligrams a day.

Milk is not only one of the most convenient ways of keeping up the calcium, it is also the form which is most readily absorbed by the body. You need not only have it with cereals, but could take it as a long, cool drink or combine it with yoghurt and fruit as a shake. Ready-made milk shakes can be bought at all supermarkets. Don't worry too much about the sugar they contain. Getting milk into the teenagers is the important thing and they can always brush their teeth afterwards. If your teenager goes off regular milk, make sure you stock up on calcium-enriched soya milk and products, and add sunflower seeds, chopped or flaked almonds and dried figs or apricots to cereals. Peanut butter on toast is good for calcium too.

Iron is also vital for growing adolescents, boys as well as girls. In a large government survey of children's eating habits it was found that all children except for older teenage boys were getting less than the recommended amount of iron. Some older girls were on very low intakes, especially those on slimming diets who also have particularly heavy menstrual losses.

The main sources of iron in the diet were found to be breakfast cereals and bread, which just goes to show how vital a meal breakfast is to the overall health of teenagers. Always try to choose breakfast cereals with added iron. A serving can supply a good 25 per cent of the day's needs. This is especially important if the teenagers don't eat much or any red meat. Having fruit or a fruit juice which contains vitamin C at breakfast will help absorption of the iron. Avoiding tea, which hinders absorption, is also a good idea.

Teenage years are the time to reinforce good eating habits and if the rest of day is often unstructured when it comes to food, breakfast can provide the one regular, well-balanced meal. Sitting down to eat it also helps establish some form of social interaction with others in the family and is a time to instil table manners. It may sound extraordinary, but breakfast may be the only meal of the day at which many teenagers have to use cutlery. Think about it. If lunch is fast food, that is normally taken straight from pack to mouth with no knife and fork required. The same goes for sandwiches and rolls, crisps, chocolate and biscuits. If supper is pizza or kebabs, the same rules apply.

It is sensible to increase fibre intakes by encouraging the eating of some wholewheat cereals, because now is the time to think about protecting against bowel cancer in later life. A diet rich in wholewheat cereals can help even from this seemingly young age. Skimmed milk and low-fat products are fine for adolescents so long as they are growing properly.

For teenagers worried about their weight, having breakfast can help stabilize things. Eating a balanced low-fat, high-carbohydrate meal before leaving home has been shown to help reduce mid-morning snacking on high-fat foods.

Getting any teenager to eat what and when they don't want to can be a battle. Sometimes there's more than one way of skinning a cat. Here are a few of the more unusual reasons I was given by teenagers for tucking into breakfast.

Joanne Seaward is thirteen. 'I sell things from the packed lunch my mum gives me at breaktime and then use the money to buy something from the van that's parked outside the school gates at lunchtime. I eat lots of breakfast so that I can last through until lunchtime, then I've just got enough to buy a hotdog and Coke, which I love.'

Nigel Roberts, who is fifteen, has similarly commercially related reasons for breakfasting before school. 'I eat as much as I can before leaving home because I'm permanently hungry. If I didn't I'd spend all my pocket money on the way to school. I spend enough of it in breaktime anyway. I don't understand how people my age can afford to skip breakfast.'

Whatever their reasons, at least both Joanne and Nigel eat breakfast. Skipping it is common among older teenage girls.

This habit is usually motivated by similar reasons as those of Katie Bruce, a slim sixteen-year-old: 'I'm always trying to be careful about what I eat. I'm worried about putting on weight even though everyone says I'm fine and shouldn't get obsessed. Skipping breakfast means I save a few hundred calories. I do get hungry but I just try to forget about it until lunchtime.'

Katie and thousands of girls like her need a quick lesson in nutrition. Studies have shown that people who miss breakfast end up being heavier than those who start the day with a high-carbohydrate, low-fat meal. These teenage girls may be keeping their weight down now, but they could be creating a habit that backfires in the future.

Singles

More and more people are opting to live the single life well into their twenties and often beyond. How many sit down to lunch or come home and cook a meal for themselves? Quick sandwiches, ready meals, take-aways and a rushed doner kebab are more likely to be chosen. It's a lucky person who can get away with continual eating on the hoof and still retain that lean physique of teenage years. Spare tyres creep up from behind, six-pack stomachs turn to beer guts and previously cellulite-free zones become pitted with deplorable dimples. Is this inevitable? No.

The question is how you can start to get things back on track. How about beginning the day with some form of structure? Breakfast offers the one opportunity at which some semblance of healthy eating can take place with incredible ease. Dr Andrew Prentice, Head of Energy Metabolism at the Dunn Nutrition Centre, puts it like this: 'There is abundant scientific evidence that low-fat diets are useful in maintaining a healthy body weight. Breakfast offers the ideal opportunity to start the day with a low-fat, high-carbohydrate meal in a highly palatable form.'

Not only can breakfast help you control your weight and stoke up on essential nutrients, it can ensure your brain's in top gear too. It's not just schoolkids whose mental performance takes a nosedive on an empty stomach. Adult breakfast-skippers show less ability to concentrate too. If you're trying to keep down a job while keeping up a social whirl, then you'd be a fool to leave home without it. If there's no time for breakfast at home or you really don't fancy it, then take it with you. Fruit, Nutrigrain bars, an individual carton of orange juice. All are completely mobile. So too are the individual cereal 'portion-paks', which can be taken along with a bowl, spoon and UHT milk to enjoy if you work behind a desk.

How about having Kids?

If you do decide to give up the young, free and single life, the chances are that sooner or later you'll be thinking of having kids. Getting into shape nutritionally is more important than you might think. Women especially should start increasing their intake of the B vitamin folic acid, which helps reduce the risk of having a baby with spina bifida. You can increase intakes by taking a 400-microgram supplement daily and by consciously eating foods such as dark green vegetables, wholemeal bread, and foods with added folic acid. Certain breakfast cereals and brands of bread like Mighty White and some supermarket own brands have extra folic acid added and carry the Health Education Authority's 'With Extra Folic Acid' flash (see page 48). This means that a typical serving will provide an extra 100 micrograms of folic acid.

Men need to shape up too. Getting enough of the antioxidant vitamins C and E and the minerals selenium and zinc is important for healthy sperm. Wholegrain cereals and wholemeal bread supply E and zinc, while citrus fruits and fruit juices are excellent for C, and brazil nuts great for selenium. Try chopping a few brazil nuts into your favourite bowl of cereal. Some, like Kellogg's Sustain, have the unique advantage of supplying 30 per cent of a man's daily zinc requirement.

Don't forget fibre too. Wholemeal bread and wholegrain cereals don't just supply useful vitamins and minerals but also give your large intestine its daily workout. It's never to late to start protecting yourself against colon cancer. And remember, the good habits you put into action now will be passed on to your kids as they grow up. See it as an investment for the future.

When the Kids have Flown

Now's the time to concentrate on taking care of yourself. If you've always put yourself in second place, then reassess. If you've always looked after your health, now isn't the time to let it slip. Keep up the good work and start by kicking the day off in the way you mean to go on.

Order some milk in. As we get older our bone density starts to fall and women especially become prone to the thinning of bones known as osteoporosis. Having a milk-and-cereal breakfast followed by a slice of toast and marmalade means you're getting a good 237 milligrams of calcium, around a quarter of your daily needs, in one go. Eating plenty of calcium-rich foods, taking regular walks and stopping smoking can all help to slow down this loss.

Don't let up on the fibre. Rates of bowel cancer rise after fifty and it's never too late to up your intakes. Cereals like All-Bran Plus and All-Bran Bite Size supply half of the daily 18-gram requirement in just one bowl. Shredded Wheat, Fibre 1 and Weetabix are other good sources. A couple of slices of wholemeal bread and an apple grated onto cereal or into yoghurt add another few grams.

Looking for the 'Extra Folic Acid' flash could stand you in good stead now since evidence strongly suggests that increasing intakes can help lower your chances of developing heart disease, men and women alike. Take a look at Chapter 6 on folic acid and heart disease to find out more.

Drinking a glass of fruit juice will do you yet more good. Rich as it is in vitamin C, you'll be helping to keep your immune system robust, not to mention your skin in fine condition too. It also helps you absorb iron from the cereals to ward off problems with anaemia. Tea has the opposite effect – it hinders iron absorption – so try to leave your cuppa for later in the day and have juice for breakfast instead.

Keep your weight in check. The last thing you want is excess blubber in your retirement. It gets in the way, slows you down, helps wear your joints out and makes you prone to both heart disease and diabetes. A balanced, low-fat, high-carbohydrate breakfast can help you control your weight.

The Sporting Life

Everyone should try to keep active. Not only does regular exercise make you feel good, it clearly helps you keep in shape by toning muscles and burning off the excess calories that could otherwise turn to fat. Whether your 'workout' involves regular walks, cycling, getting down to the gym or thrashing around on a football pitch, what you eat can help you sustain an active lifestyle.

To exercise you need energy. The muscles' main sources of energy, or fuel, are carbohydrates and fats. The amount used depends on the type of activity you do, how hard you do it and how long you do it for. Short sharp bursts of activity, such as sprinting for a football, are fuelled by carbohydrate. Longer duration activities, such as swimming, cycling or running, use a mix of carbohydrate and fat. The longer you exercise, the more fat is used.

Most of us have huge reserves of fat even if we aren't exactly overweight. If we are carrying around extra fat then we have even larger stores. Either way, under normal sporting circumstances there's no chance that we're going to exhaust supplies. With carbohydrate stores it's a different story. We store carbohydrate in our liver and muscles but only in quite small amounts. Each time we do something active the stores need topping up to make sure there's enough for next time round.

Think about it. Have you ever embarked on a mad week of keep fit? Have you been to several aerobics classes, gone out for walks and generally dashed around only to find that each time you go to a class you feel worse, not better? This is more than likely down to not eating enough carbohydrate between sessions to refill your muscle stores. It's like trying to run a car long distances on a single tank of petrol. The petrol level goes down until eventually, if you don't fill up, you come to a grinding halt. The body is no different. Active people need plenty of carbohydrates.

A diet based around starchy carbohydrates is recommended for everyone. When you're active, it's even more important to follow this advice. A really sporty man or youngster eating a daily 3,000 calories would need to make sure that he ate 450 grams of carbohydrate every day (in other words, 1,800 of the calories would come from carbohydrates). A sporty woman eating 2,000 calories needs about 300 grams a day (1,200-calories' worth).

For recreationally active women who manage to exercise three times a week, about 5 grams of carbohydrate per kilogram of body weight is fine. For someone weighing 55 kilos that's 275 grams of carbohydrate a day. If you think about the kind of things you can eat at breakfast, you'll see how easy it is to boost your carbs at the first meal of the day.

Foods supplying 50 grams of Carbohydrate

50 grams of breakfast cereal with skimmed milk
3 slices of toast
2 bread rolls
1 banana sandwich (2 slices of bread and 1 banana)
1 bagel
4–5 oatcakes
3 slices of malt loaf
1 1/2 wholemeal muffins
4 toasted crumpets
2 Nutrigrain bars

After breakfast it's important to maintain good carbohydrate intakes throughout the day by basing meals around starchy foods such as rice, pasta, bread or potatoes. Add to this some protein such as chicken, fish, a little red meat or plenty of pulses, and include several servings of vegetables and fruits for an overall balance to your diet. It is also important to eat some carbohydrate food within two hours of exercising, since this is the time when muscles are able to refuel at their fastest.

Keeping up the Fluid

When you're active it's also essential to make sure you drink plenty of fluids. We all need a good 1.5 litres of water a day to keep us ticking over. Add to this another litre of water for every hour of activity you undertake. By the time you are thirsty you are already dehydrated, and being dehydrated makes you feel tired and less like keeping up the exercise. Drinking during and straight after exercise helps to maintain a good fluid balance.

What about the Protein?

Contrary to popular belief, to gain muscle you don't need to eat loads of protein foods and take protein supplement drinks. Even serious sports people don't need more than 1.5 grams of protein per kilo of body weight each day. This would mean an average 70-kilo man needing 105 grams a day, which he would get in a pint of milk, a bowl of cereal and two slices of toast for breakfast, a large tuna sandwich for lunch, some chicken and pasta for dinner and a fromage frais. Most men, however, need only around half this amount, which is easily obtained in a mixed diet.

For an average active woman, 45 grams of protein a day is enough, and for a really sporty one this increases to 1.2 grams per kilo of body weight. A sporty woman of 55 kilos would therefore need about 80 grams, which, again, you easily get from a normal mixed diet.

Chapter 14

How the Celebrities breakfast

Bruce Forsyth, entertainer

Half a cantaloupe melon
Bran Flakes with a handful of raisins
Tea

'My breakfast is always the same, unless I'm feeling really reckless and add a few Cinnamon Toasties! I believe in eating lots of fruit during the morning and it's just part of my routine. I get incredibly grumpy if my melon isn't just how I like it – sweet and not hard. I take garlic tablets and cod-liver-oil capsules at breakfast-time. You have to look after yourself in this business since it's physically and mentally demanding. I had my most memorable breakfasts when my beautiful wife Winnalia and I were on honeymoon in Mawi, Hawaii. We would breakfast on exotic fruits watching the American version of Mr and Mrs, which was racier than our programme here. We'd see which questions we got right and have a good laugh. Then it was off to the beach or race course for the rest of the day.'

Ulrika Jonsson, television presenter

Live yoghurt
Bran Flakes with prunes
Semi-skimmed milk
Coffee

'My breakfasts have changed over the years. In Sweden when I was a child we had 'Fil' yoghurt based on sour milk, along with muesli and cold sausage and ham. This was always washed down with a gorgeous chocolate milk drink which is still my major weakness. I don't go anywhere without my tub of Nesquick. I'm ashamed to admit I used to have three breakfasts when I was doing TVAM. Toast with butter and marmalade at 4.30 a.m. in the make-up room, cereal at the 7.30 break and a full fry-up with everyone in the canteen at 9.30. Our lives revolved around breakfast so I really went for it until I realized I was ballooning and had to cut back. While I was pregnant I ate All-Bran to be sure I got plenty of fibre. After my son was born I sometimes didn't have a chance to grab anything at all. I'm back into the swing now and eating my usual breakfast of prunes and yoghurt.'

Graham Cowdray, Kent County cricket player

'What I have for breakfast depends where we are in the cricket season. Come October when I'm getting into shape we tend to stay in a lot of hotels. It takes all my willpower not to dig into a traditional breakfast – I resist and go for something more continental. I always have lots of wholewheat cereal to get my bran in so it would either be All-Bran or Fruit 'n' Fibre with a chopped banana. Along with this I have to have industrial-strength coffee. I'm a coffee fiend and probably drink too much. These days the fitness tests we undergo are very strict so we have to be fit. That's why come the time for playing I take having a good breakfast seriously. The best breakfasts I can remember having were at the Jamaica Inn Hotel in Jamaica where my wife Maxine and I would sit on our balcony being served endless amount of fruits – and of course coffee!'

Tim Henman, tennis player

David Felgate, Henman's coach, says: 'The key is balance and one way to get this into Tim's routine is at least to start the day with a good breakfast. Usually it's fortified cereal with extra vitamins and minerals. If you're not getting them in your diet then eating them when they've been added to other foods is a good idea.'

Frank Bruno, retired boxer

Crunchy Nut Corn Flakes with milk

'Although I'm not boxing any more, I still like to keep fit. I train every day and have a healthy diet. I know breakfast is really important. It gives me the best start to the day, keeping my energy levels high. I never forget to have my bowl of Crunchy Nut Corn Flakes in the morning.'

Lord Archer, author

Corn Flakes with whole milk and raspberries
2 boiled eggs
Glass of milk

'I often have breakfast at the Savoy and this would be the typical order. Once when I was breakfasting there with my long-time friend and renowned barrister Lord Alexander, we ordered 'kippers' and were dismayed to find we were served only one each. I was so livid I threatened to sue until I discovered that Lord Alexander had sided with the Savoy. Apparently because the discrepancy between what was on the menu and what we were actually served had been there for fifteen years, the law of precedence meant they were within their rights. Now I have boiled eggs instead, as a matter of principle. If I'm at home then it's Corn Flakes and any fruit that happens to be in the fridge. I'm naturally a lark so when I'm writing a book I'm up at 6.00 a.m., write to 8.00 and have my Corn Flakes then.'

Katie Boyle, personality

Half a grapefruit
Raisin Splits with Canderel and skimmed milk
Lemon tea

'If I don't eat in the morning I'm violently ill and can't do a full day's work. On Sundays I have hot Marks & Spencer's Seed Batch Loaf with butter and peach jam. The bread's so full of seeds it should be for the sparrows. Unfortunately my appetite is larger than a sparrow's and I eat far too much.'

Clare Francis, crime writer

Vegetable stir-fry
English breakfast tea

'I don't mind if people think my breakfast is odd. Personally I can't understand how anyone could possibly eat pig for breakfast. If I miss breakfast I'm flagging by midday. I like having vegetables first thing in the morning because they fill me up but don't weigh me down when I'm writing. Sometimes I have an avocado salad instead. I avoid bread or rice since both are rather heavy.'

Nic Baker, world-class English windsurfer

Muesli with low-fat milk
or
Baked beans on toast

'I've had my diet overhauled by personal trainer, Torje Eike. He's recommended these breakfasts, which I stick to. He's tried to get me to have yoghurt on my muesli but there are limits. On race days windsurfers are at the beach by 8.30 a.m. testing the water for an hour. Between then and 10.00 a.m. I manage a few bananas, then we do about twelve races during the day what with the heats and rounds. It's all very energy-intensive.'

Roger Black, athlete

Sustain or All-Bran with milk
Protein shake with 2 eggs

'There's no doubt in my mind that breakfast is the most important meal of the day. To get my carbohydrate and protein balance right I start with a bowl of Sustain or All-Bran with milk. This is followed by a protein shake. You have to make time for it, it's an essential part of the day.'

Phil de Glanville, rugby player

3 Shredded Wheat with semi-skimmed milk
Toast

'We were taught by Rex Hazeldene from Loughborough University about the importance of diet on performance. Rugby players are notoriously bad about eating and drinking. There might be some basic knowledge but not much pre-match planning. I don't think there's a very good understanding of just how much difference it makes. I always start the day with three Shredded Wheat with semi-skimmed milk – skimmed is just too horrible. I sometimes have toast if I'm not in too much of a hurry.'

Jonathon Edwards, long-jumper

Cereal with semi-skimmed milk
Wholemeal toast and Marmite
Coffee

'I try to have 60 per cent of my energy by lunchtime, which means having a good breakfast, usually cereal and toast. I've had nutritional advice and have changed the timing of my meals to improve my insulin balance throughout the day.'

Va'aiga Tuigamala, rugby player

'I fully endorse the idea that you should breakfast like a king. It's the most important meal of the day for me. I'm fussy about it. I eat before 8.00 a.m. and it usually consists of bread and fresh fruit. I keep an eye on my weight every morning because I know at the weekend there are forty thousand people in the crowd doing it for me!'

Chapter 15

The Breakfast Quiz

1. At the beginning of the century a fry-up was considered a typical English breakfast. How many of us now regularly tuck into bacon and eggs?

   i) 13 per cent   ii) 20 per cent   iii) 30 per cent

answer: i) 13 per cent

2. Which is the world's best-selling breakfast cereal?

answer: Kellogg's Corn Flakes. In 1996 sales reached £99 million worldwide

3. You would need to eat four bananas to get the same amount of fibre as a bowl of All Bran. True or False?

answer: False, you actually need to eat nine!

4. In which country is Snap! Crackle! and Pop! known as Cric! Crac! Croc!?

   i) Italy   ii) France   iii) Germany

answer: ii) France

5. Which country eats the most cereal per person in the world?

   i) America   ii) Ireland   iii) England

answer: ii) Ireland. They chomp their way through the equivalent of 7.7 kilos (17 pounds) of cereal per person every year.

6. Breakfast helps children do better in their schoolwork by improving their concentration. True or False?

answer: True

7. John Harvey and Will Kellogg invented Corn Flakes, but what did they also invent?

   i) Peanut butter   ii) Pop Corn   iii) Crispbreads

answer: i) Peanut butter

8. In which American town were Corn Flakes first invented?

   i) Boston   ii) Baltimore   iii) Battle Creek

answer: iii) Battle Creek

9. What's the name of the world's only 'talking' cereal?

answer: Rice Krispies

10. A breakfast of fried egg, fried bread and two rashers of bacon contains 42 grams of fat, and a bowl of cereal with semi-skimmed milk around 5 grams. True or False?

answer: True

11. Eating more fibre may help reduce the risk of colon cancer and breast cancer. True or False?

answer: True

12. Take a guess which country wakes up to noodles, rice, pastries and sour milk?

   i) Korea   ii) Columbia   iii) Poland

answer: i) Korea

13. What is the total amount of fat per day an average man and an average woman should be aiming to consume?
   i) 90g men, 70g women
   ii) 100g men, 80g women
   iii) 110g men, 90g women

answer: i) 90g men, 70g women

14. Milk, such as that you pour on your cereal, is especially good for your bones. True or False?

answer: True. Milk's high content of calcium is particularly good for building strong bones

15. The iron you find in fortified breakfast cereals is better absorbed when you have it with:
   i) A cup of tea
   ii) A cup of coffee
   iii) A glass of orange juice

answer: iii) A glass of orange juice because it contains vitamin C

16. Some cereals have extra folic acid added. This seems to help reduce the risk of which of the following problems?
   i) Having a baby with spina bifida
   ii) Having heart disease
   iii) Fracturing your bones

answer: Both i) and ii)

17. In tests, people who ate 60 grams (two bowls) of breakfast cereal a day without following any other dietary advice lost weight. True or False?

answer: True. The group of women studied lost an average of 1.5 kilograms over a twelve-week period when following this advice. Those women who were a little overweight at the start of the twelve weeks lost more.

18. A portion of sweetened breakfast cereal contains the same amount of sugar as you'd find in a medium-sized apple. True or false?

answer: True. There's about 12 grams, a couple of teaspoons, in each

19. What do Lord Archer, Bruce Forsyth and Ulrika Jonsson have in common?

answer: They all start their day with a bowl of cereal

20. What does Frank Bruno usually have for breakfast?

answer: Crunchy Nut Corn Flakes

Chapter 16

The 28-Day Zest-for-Life Diet Plan

Let's get one thing clear. Losing weight is not easy. It needs willpower, motivation and long-term commitment. That's the bad news. Now here's some good news. At last it's been shown that there's absolutely no point in putting your bodies through the agonies of quick-fix 1,000-calorie diets. Anyone who's tried them will know that these starvation rations are impossible to stick to for long. They leave you feeling hungry, tired, de-motivated and, once you finally crack under the strain, likely to pile all the weight back on in a few days of gorging. If this routine sounds familiar, don't feel bad about it. That kind of response is completely natural. You haven't failed, and it's not your fault. Your body has simply taken over with its survival instinct. It needs more food!

With this diet plan we're taking a more realistic approach. No starvation, no false hopes. You won't lose a stone in a week but you will, if you keep on track, shed a good two pounds of fat a week. Doesn't sound much, I know. But think about it. Two pounds a week is half a stone a month while you're still able to drink alcohol, eat chocolates and feel full. Keep going for two more months and you'll have burnt off one and a half stone; do it for six and some three stone could have vanished into thin air.

All of that just by making changes to how you eat. Add a bit of regular exercise and the whole process gets speeded up.

The Sums

If you have more than three stone to lose, eat 1,500 calories a day. That may sound a lot, but it's probably a good 1,000 less than you currently eat. People invariably underestimate their daily calorie intake. I do, even though as a nutritionist you'd think I'd get it right. It's not that I'm trying to kid myself, it's just incredibly hard to remember every single thing I've chewed my way through. A bar of chocolate mid-morning, those biscuits with coffee, that packet of crisps at 4 o'clock.

The other thing to remember is that the more weight you're carrying around, the higher your metabolic rate, which means you need to cut back less than a smaller person in order to start burning fat. A woman who weighs 16 stone, for example, could easily be burning 2,600–2,800 calories a day. Cutting back to 1,500 would mean 1,000 fewer calories per day, or 7,000 fewer per week, which is equivalent to 2 pounds of fat.

For people with less than 2 stone to lose it's advisable to try the 1,300-calorie-a-day option. If you weigh around 12 stone you're probably burning up about 2,200 calories per day. Eat any less than 1,300 and you'll be entering that starvation area, which will feel like hell.

To help shift the fat it's vital to get active. Not buying a skimpy bit of Lycra and heading for the gym, but incorporating exercise into your life by taking regular walks, cycling indoors or out if you've got a bike and using the stairs instead of lifts. If you can swim and have a pool nearby then take the plunge. Think about taking lessons if you haven't learnt before. If all of these sound dull, consider yoga, Pilates, kick boxing, dancing – anything, but just get off your bum and start moving.

How to use the Diet

There are sixteen breakfasts to choose from, each of which supplies around 300 calories. You can have the same one every day, follow them in order, or just mix and match as you fancy. Some are intended for eating at home, others are mobile to fit in with your routine.

Then comes lunch, which needs to be 400 calories in total. There are twenty-eight recipes to choose from, plus a few quick lunch ideas too. The lunch suggestions supply around 300 or 350 calories each. To those which are 300 calories, add a food from 100-calorie extras to make it up to 400. With the 350-calorie lunches add one of the 50-calorie extras to make it up to

400. You can follow the lunches in order – there's a four-week supply – or pick and choose the ones you prefer or find easier to prepare. If you live life on the run, choose any of the ready-made sandwiches with calories listed from the supermarkets and large chemists. Opt for reduced-fat versions and don't go above 400. If you find 300-calorie versions you know you have another 100 to use up as before.

Dinners, as with lunches, should supply 400 calories. The suggestions here – again, there are twenty-eight recipes, plus quick meal ideas – supply around 300 or 350 calories. Choose the ones you like and make up the extra calories from the 50- or 100-calorie suggestions. A few of the more substantial dinners contain 400 calories, which means there's no room for extras. For those of you who can't stand the thought of cooking or just don't have time, then you can choose ready-meals up to 400 calories. If you choose 300-calorie ones you have 100 extra to play with, as before.

By having 300 calories at breakfast and 400 each at lunch and dinner you will be getting 1,100 in total. Add to this half of a pint of skimmed milk a day for teas and coffees to bring this up to 1,200.

For those with two stone or less to lose make this up to 1,300 calories a day by choosing any one of the 100-calorie options or two of the 50-calorie options.

For those with more than 2 stone to lose, make it up to 1,500 by choosing three 100-calorie extras or six 50-calorie extras, at least 100 of which should be fruit.

Don't forget, if you are a woman of childbearing age, take an extra 400 micrograms of folic acid a day. Check with your GP that it's OK to follow a healthy eating plan and to start getting more active through regularly taking up walking, dancing, swimming or an activity of your choice.

There are really just two rules: don't skip breakfast and enjoy it!

Breakfasts

A tasty, filling, nutritious breakfast doesn't need ages to prepare. The fastest breakfast of all has to be a quick bowl of cereal. No cooking, no mess. All you need is a bowl and a spoon. If you've got a little more time, grate over an apple or chop in a banana. For days when you have more time, try whipping up one of the other ideas. Whatever you do, make sure you eat something before leaving home. If this is completely impossible then look at the mobile breakfasts. These are ideas for people on the move or who breakfast at their desk. If you find it tricky to organize even this before leaving home, then don't forget you can buy a full range of Kellogg's Portion-Paks to leave at work and eat once you get there. Use fresh skimmed milk, or keep UHT milk at hand, or even skimmed milk powder which you can make up each day to enjoy your breakfast when it fits into your schedule. A few minutes' planning can make or break your day. There's no excuse!

Each breakfast idea serves one, apart from the Bran Fruit Loaf.

Five-minute Wonders

1. Quick 'n' Fit
40 grams of Special K served with a sliced banana and cold skimmed milk.

300 calories   1 gram of fat

2. Fibre Provider
40 grams of Bran Flakes or Fruit 'n' Fibre topped with 100 grams of drained tinned peaches (use the ones in natural juice). Cover with cold skimmed milk and serve with a cool glass of grapefruit juice.

300 calories   1 gram of fat

3. The Chocolate Fix
Smother 40 grams of Choco Krispies with cold skimmed milk. (If you fancy it, mix some orange zest into the milk for an added buzz.) Follow this with 200 ml fresh orange juice.

300 calories   1 gram of fat

4. *The Country Crunch*
Grab the box of Crunchy Nut Corn Flakes and serve yourself 40 grams. Quickly grate over a washed apple. Top with a tablespoon of yoghurt and serve with 200 ml cold skimmed milk.

272 calories   2 grams of fat

5. *Quick Croissant*
Stir a teaspoon of honey into a plain yoghurt and eat while you are heating up a croissant. Enjoy the croissant with a large teaspoon of jam of your choice.

300 calories   11 grams of fat

6. *Fresh 'n' Fruity*
Use three of your favourite fruits – some fresh, some canned if it's easier. Why not try a chopped banana with canned apricots in natural juice and a freshly grated crisp apple? Top with a 150-gram carton of low-fat fruit yoghurt of your choice.

300 calories   2 grams of fat

7. *French Toast*
Leave 2 slices of bread out overnight. In the morning whisk 1 egg with a pinch of cinnamon, brown sugar and nutmeg. Dip the slices of bread into the egg mix and fry in a non-stick pan oiled with a single spray of Fry Light. Cook for 2–3 minutes each side. While still hot, top with 2 tablespoons of very low-fat fromage frais and some slices of fresh apple.

300 calories   8 grams of fat

8. *Microwave Magic Porridge*
Mix 40 grams of porridge oats with 140 ml skimmed milk and 40 grams of ready-to eat-apricots, figs or sultanas. Microwave for 1 1/2 minutes on full power. Stir and allow to stand for 1 minute. Eat with a tablespoon of low-fat fromage frais and a teaspoon of honey.

300 calories   4 grams of fat

9. Egg-White and Smoked Haddock Flat Omelette

Whisk up 3 egg whites and season with salt and pepper. Heat up a non-stick frying pan and spray with a shot of Fry Light. Pour in the egg whites and shake the pan well. Place 50 grams of flaked haddock on the egg whites. Put under the grill for 3 minutes and turn out on to the serving plate. Eat with 2 slices of toast and a grilled tomato.

300 calories   3 grams of fat

10. Special Salmon Bagel

Cut a plain bagel in half and spread with one tablespoon of very low-fat fromage frais. Divide 25 grams of smoked salmon between each bagel half and sprinkle with lemon juice. Grind some black pepper over and eat with a glass of chilled vegetable or fruit juice alongside.

300 calories   3 grams of fat

11. Apple and Date Oat Flakes

Pour 50 grams of oat flakes into a bowl and stir in 30 grams of chopped dates. Grate over an apple and pour in some cold skimmed milk. Top with a tablespoon of virtually fat-free fromage frais or yoghurt.

300 calories   2 grams of fat

12. Grill-up

Grill a rasher of bacon and a small low-fat sausage along with 2 large mushrooms and 1 tomato. Serve on 2 slices of toast (no butter or margarine). Accompany with a small glass of fruit juice.

300 calories   11 grams of fat

Mobile Breakfasts

If you just can't face breakfast first thing then don't skip it altogether. Remember, skippers end up weighing more than breakfast eaters.

13. Shake it Up

Stock up ready-made milk shakes such as Break Time chocolate-flavour drink (available in ASDA), Frijj banana flavour, Marks & Spencer Kool Chocolate Shake or Onken drinking yoghurt. All provide around 300 calories in their 500 ml serving. Alternatively have 250 ml cold semi-skimmed milk plus a large banana.

300 calories   2 grams of fat

14. Nutrigrain Bar

Take a strawberry, apple or blueberry Nutrigrain bar along with a banana and individual carton of orange juice to work with you. Eat when you can mid-morning.

300 calories   4 grams of fat

15. Mango and Mint Whip

Drain 150 grams of canned mango and blend with 2 tablespoons of low-fat yoghurt. Add a few chopped mint leaves. Pour into a plastic container with a lid. Once ready to eat, crumb over a Nutrigrain bar to give a lovely texture.

300 calories   4 grams of fat

16. Bran Fruit Loaf

Put 100 grams of All-Bran, 150 grams of sugar and 275 grams of dried mixed fruit into a basin and mix them well together. Stir in 300 ml of skimmed milk and leave to stand for half an hour. Sieve in 100 grams of flour, mixing well, and pour the mixture into a well-greased 900-gram loaf tin. Bake in a moderate oven (180oC/gas 4) for about 1 hour. Turn out of the tin immediately and allow to cool. Cut into 8 slices. Pack a slice in foil and take an apple or small banana to eat with it. (Keeps for 3 days.)

240 calories   0.6 gram of fat

Lunches

Each recipe or suggestion here serves one. Baked potatoes should weigh between 120 and 150 grams. Slices of bread are from a medium-sized loaf.

1. Salmon Spread Bagel

Mix 50 grams of flaked canned salmon with 50 grams of very low-fat fromage frais, a teaspoon each of lemon juice and horseradish sauce, some black pepper, and chopped fresh coriander if you have it. Split the bagel in half and cover both cut surfaces with a layer of finely sliced cucumber. Pile the salmon spread on top, grind some more black pepper over and serve with extra cucumber cut into sticks.

350 calories   6 grams of fat

2. Mexican Bean Spread

Take 2 heaped tablespoons of low-fat yoghurt and stir in a good pinch each of ground cumin and chilli powder, plus some black pepper. Blend or thoroughly mash this with 100 grams of drained canned red kidney beans. Mix in a handful of chopped fresh coriander leaves. Slice a tomato and shred some lettuce. Split a pitta bread and fill with the spread and salad.

306 calories   5 grams of fat

3. Avocado Dip with Rice Cakes

Mash or blend 100 grams of canned peas with a small avocado that has been peeled and the stone removed. Finely dice a tomato and a small onion and stir into the pea and avocado mixture along with a tablespoon of lemon juice, a dash of Worcester sauce, a pinch each of cayenne pepper and chilli powder, and some freshly ground black pepper. Spread this reduced-fat guacamole over 4 rice cakes and eat with carrot batons.

350 calories   18 grams of fat

4. Peanut Butter Crumpets

Mix 1 tablespoon of peanut butter with 1 tablespoon of low-fat fromage frais. Spread over 3 toasted crumpets. Top the crumpets with slices of cucumber for extra moisture and serve with slices of apple.

400 calories   10 grams of fat

5. Cottage Coleslaw Jacket

Either use a 200-gram serving of ready-made reduced-calorie coleslaw or make your own using finely shredded cabbage and onion, a grated carrot and 2 tablespoons of reduced-fat salad cream. Mix into this 100 grams of cottage cheese and use to fill a medium-sized baked jacket potato.

300 calories   6 grams of fat

6. Chilli Fried Eggs on Toast

Toast 2 slices of bread from frozen. Once they've popped up, cool and toast again to maximize crispness. Heat a non-stick pan, spray with a shot of Fry Light, then crack in 1 egg and gently fry for 4 minutes. Meanwhile, cut a tomato in half, spray with Fry Light and grill. Add to the frying pan half a chopped fresh red chilli and a sprinkling of garlic salt. When the egg is ready, place on one slice of toast, with the grilled tomato on the other. Sprinkle with some chopped fresh parsley.

300 calories   5 grams of fat

7. Herby Scrambled Eggs

In a bowl beat an egg well, then add 2 tablespoons of skimmed milk and a sprinkling of garlic salt. Whisk to combine. Put some mushrooms on to grill. Prepare 2 slices of toast. Heat a non-stick pan, spray with a shot of Fry Light and pour in the eggs. Stir well over a very low heat until the eggs are softly scrambled then stir in some freshly chopped parsley, tarragon and chervil (use fresh herbs, if you can). Serve the eggs on one slice of toast and the mushrooms on the other.

300 calories   8 grams of fat

8. Sweetcorn Fritters

Blend 40 grams of canned sweetcorn with 1 teaspoon of mustard, 1 tablespoon of plain flour and 2 tablespoons of skimmed milk. Then add another 20 grams of sweetcorn and leave them whole in the mix. Take 2 egg whites and whisk until soft peaks form. Add a pinch of salt, then fold into the sweetcorn mix. Heat up a non-stick pan, add a single shot of Fry Light and drop spoonfuls of the mix into the pan. Cook for 3 minutes each side, then serve with two sliced tomatoes topped with shredded basil and a 70-gram chunk of fresh white or granary bread.

300 calories   3 grams of fat

9. Caesar Light

Toast 2 slices of wholemeal bread. Cut one slice into cubes, allow to cool then rub a clove of peeled garlic over the surfaces. Meanwhile, shred a good handful of Cos lettuce and put in a bowl with 80 grams of diced cooked chicken and 2 tablespoons of Weight Watchers Caesar-style dressing. Toss in the cubes of toast, mix together, and then arrange 10 grams of Parmesan shavings (or sprinkle over 10 grams of grated Parmesan) and a chopped canned anchovy, if you like them, over the top. Serve with the extra slice of toast.

300 calories   9 grams of fat

10. Pawpaw and Cottage Cheese Toast

Put 120 grams of low-fat cottage cheese into a bowl, add 1 teaspoon of Dijon mustard and 1/2 teaspoon of grain mustard, and mix well. Scoop out the flesh from a small pawpaw (also known as papaya). Mash with a little lemon juice and spread over two slices of cooled toast. Top with the cottage cheese.

300 calories   4 grams of fat

11. BLT Whopper

Spread 3 slices of bread with reduced-fat salad cream, spreading one of the slices on both sides. Place a slice of bread on a plate with the salad-cream side up. Lay a rasher of grilled chopped bacon and some shredded lettuce on it. Place the doubly-spread slice on top and cover with slices of tomato. Grind some black pepper over and finish with the third slice of bread. Insert 4 cocktail sticks and cut into 4 triangles.

320 calories   12 grams of fat

12. Hummus with Crispbreads
Into 50 grams of reduced-fat hummus mix 30 grams of fat-free fromage frais, a dash of Worcester sauce and some lemon juice. Spread over 50 grams of crispbread (such as Ryvita, Harvest Slims or Harvest Wheats). Serve with piles of carrot and cucumber sticks.

300 calories   3 grams of fat

13. Prawn Mayo Potatoes
Bake or microwave a medium-sized potato (160 grams). Spoon the potato from the skin and mash with some lemon juice, setting the skins aside. Mix together 1 tablespoon of low-fat Thousand Island dressing with 1 tablespoon of plain yoghurt, then stir in 60 grams of cooked prawns and some freshly ground black pepper. Combine with the potato and return to the potato skins. Serve with green salad dressed with fat-free vinaigrette.

350 calories   5 grams of fat

14. Salad Niçoise
Boil 2 potatoes (120 grams), allow to cool then dice. Blanch 50 grams of French beans and allow to cool. Mix the potatoes and beans with lots of shredded lettuce, a chopped tomato, 100 grams of flaked tuna (the kind that's canned in brine) and 2 tablespoons of fat-free vinaigrette. Arrange 2 halved olives and 2 anchovies on top.

300 calories   12 grams of fat

15. Hot Egg and Ham Muffins
Split a muffin and toast both sides. Lay a slice of ham on each surface. On one place a grilled tomato, on the other a poached egg.

350 calories   13 grams of fat

16. Quick Kipper Kedgeree

Take 50 grams of kipper (frozen ones are an easy option). Cook according to packet instructions, and keep the cooking liquid. Meanwhile cook 50 grams of rice, drain and allow to cool; hardboil an egg, allow to cool then finely chop or grate. Heat a non-stick frying pan, spray with a single shot of Fry Light and sauté half a chopped onion with 1 teaspoon of curry powder. Add the cooked rice, kipper and egg and a squeeze of fresh lemon juice and cook for 4 minutes. Serve with chopped fresh parsley, freshly ground black pepper and a lemon wedge to squeeze over.

380 calories   14 grams of fat

17. Pâté Crumpets

Toast 2 crumpets and spread with a total of 40 grams of reduced-fat pâté. Top with slices of tomato and freshly ground black pepper. Serve with a salad made from a grated carrot mixed with 2 tablespoons of fat-free vinaigrette, 2 teaspoons of raisins and a sprinkling of poppy seeds.

300 calories   9 grams of fat

18. Russian Salad

Hardboil an egg, allow to cool then quarter. Boil 2 potatoes (120 grams), allow to cool then chop. Cook 2 tablespoons of frozen peas and 50 grams of green beans, then allow both to cool. Meanwhile, dice 50 grams of chicken or ham, finely chop 1 carrot, and mix 1 tablespoon of plain yoghurt with 1 tablespoon of reduced-fat salad cream. Combine all the ingredients except the egg with the dressing. Garnish the salad with the quartered egg.

350 calories   14 grams of fat

19. Crabmeat Pitta Pockets

Mix 2 tablespoons of low-fat plain yoghurt with 1 tablespoon of low-fat Thousand Island dressing. Combine 80 grams of flaked canned crabmeat with a chopped spring onion, a little grated ginger (it's easier to grate if it comes from the freezer) and half a red pepper, diced. Pour over the dressing and toss to combine. Sprinkle a handful of fresh or canned and drained beansprouts with a little soy sauce and stuff into pitta bread. Put the crab mixture on top.

350 calories   5 grams of fat

20. Blue Cheese Butter Beans

Combine 100 grams of canned, drained butter beans with 50 ml (3 1/2 tablespoons) plain yoghurt, 1 tablespoon of fat-free Creamy Ranch Blue dressing (Kraft), a chopped spring onion, 40 grams of chopped ham and some chives. Serve piled on top of lettuce with large slice of granary bread.

300 calories   7 grams of fat

21. Chicken Couscous Salad

Heat a non-stick frying pan, spray with a single shot of Fry Light and pour in 65 grams of couscous. Let it roast for 4 minutes, stirring well, then pour in 125 ml vegetable stock made with a cube. Cover and leave to rest. Combine 50 grams of canned, drained chickpeas with half a red pepper, diced, a pinch of chopped parsley and the juice of 1 lemon. When the couscous has absorbed the stock, fluff with a fork then combine with the chickpea mixture. Transfer to a plate and garnish with 50 grams of cooked diced chicken. Scatter with plenty of chopped parsley and a few black olives.

350 calories   6 grams of fat

22. Cheese and Peach Malt Loaf

Spread 2 slices of malt loaf with a total of 50 grams of 'light' or reduced-fat cream cheese. Slice up a fresh peach or use 70 grams of well-drained canned peaches, and place on top.

300 calories   10 grams of fat

23. Smoked Turkey and Watercress Sandwich

Spread 2 slices of wholemeal or white bread with 1 teaspoon of reduced-fat salad cream. Fill the sandwich with 50 grams of smoked turkey or chicken, a sliced tomato and some watercress.

300 calories   6 grams of fat

24. *Barbecue Bean Rarebit*
Toast 2 thick slices of wholemeal bread and spread with 20 grams of Dairylea or Laughing Cow cheese spread. Heat up a small can of barbecue beans (135 grams) and divide between the slices. Garnish with fresh parsley, if you have some.

350 calories   8 grams of fat

25. *Mushroom Soufflé Omelette*
Heat a small frying pan or omelette pan, spray with Fry Light and sauté 2 chopped mushrooms until soft. Meanwhile, separate the yolks and whites of 2 eggs. Beat the yolks and whisk the whites until stiff. Fold together along with 2 tablespoons of hot water, a pinch of thyme and a little Dijon mustard. Pour into the hot pan with the mushrooms, cook for 3–4 minutes, then finish under a hot grill for 2 minutes. Garnish with chopped fresh parsley and serve with a warm, medium-sized roll.

300 calories   15 grams of fat

26. *Very Fast Tomato Pasta*
Cook 75 grams of spaghetti or other pasta in lots of boiling, salted water. Meanwhile, heat up 100 grams of low-fat tomato-style pasta sauce, such as Paul Newman's Sockarooni or Dolmio Light. Once the pasta is cooked, drain and add to the sauce. Toss, transfer to a dish and sprinkle with a teaspoon of grated Parmesan. Serve with a big green salad with fat-free vinaigrette.

300 calories   3 grams of fat

27. *Walnut Peach Jackets*
Bake or microwave a medium-sized baking potato. Split open, spoon out the potato flesh and mix it with 1 teaspoon of lemon juice, some freshly ground black pepper, 60 grams of low-fat

cottage cheese, a chopped peach and 10 grams of chopped walnuts. Pile it back into the potato skin, and serve a green salad with fat-free vinaigrette alongside.

350 calories   8 grams of fat

28. Feta Ciabatta

Crumble 50 grams of feta cheese into a bowl and mix in a chopped tomato, some chopped leek and a tablespoon of reduced-calorie salad cream. Split open a ciabatta roll and fill with shredded lettuce and the feta salad.

300 calories   12 grams of fat

Dinners

Each recipe or suggestion here serves two, unless otherwise stated. The calorie and fat counts are per person. Baked potatoes should weigh between 120 and 150 grams, and slices of bread are to come from a medium-sized loaf.

1. Stir-fry Vegetables with Bean Curd and Cashews

De-seed and slice 1 small red and 1 small yellow pepper and cut into 5cm strips. Cut 100 grams of broccoli on the diagonal into the same size strips making sure the stalky bits are very thin. Top and tail 100 grams of mangetout and slice 4 spring onions into rounds. Set the prepared vegetables aside on a plate. Peel and grate 3cm of ginger (from frozen ideally – it's easier to grate) and crush a large clove of garlic. Cut 100 grams of bean curd into small squares, and crush 1 tablespoon of cashew nuts. Cook 200 grams of noodles according to packet instructions. Heat 1 tablespoon of sesame or vegetable oil in a wok or heavy frying pan until very hot. Add the ginger and garlic and toss for 10 seconds. Add the bean curd and fry for 1 minute. Remove and set aside. Add all the vegetables plus the crushed cashew nuts to the hot wok and stir-fry for 1–2 minutes. Stir in 1 tablespoon of sherry or stock and 1 tablespoon rich soy sauce. Return the bean curd, ginger and garlic to the wok, stir carefully for a few seconds, then serve with the cooked, drained noodles.

300 calories   8 grams of fat

2. Braised Pork in Cider Vinegar Sauce

Heat a large heavy pan and spray with a shot of Fry Light. Add 250 grams of extra lean pork fillets, turn them until browned and then remove and set aside. Add another shot of Fry Light to the pan, then a large, chopped onion and cook until the onion is browned. Pour in 250 ml medium-sweet cider and 150 ml cider vinegar, or, if you don't have these, 350 ml of well-seasoned stock. Return the pork fillets, season with salt and pepper and add a sprig of fresh thyme and a bay leaf. Bring to a simmer, then set the lid slightly askew and cook for 1 hour until meat is tender and the sauce reduced. Serve with 300 grams of minted new potatoes and lightly steamed, shredded red cabbage.

300 calories   5 grams of fat

3. Grilled Garlic Ginger Chicken

Mix 2 tablespoons of lemon juice with 1 large, crushed clove of garlic, either 2 teaspoons of grated fresh or frozen ginger or 1 teaspoon of powdered ginger, and a pinch each of chilli and cumin powder. Place 2 boneless, skinned 150-gram chicken breasts in a shallow dish and coat with the lemon and garlic mix. Leave for 15 minutes in the fridge. Make 225 ml of stock with a vegetable stock cube, a few shakes of Tabasco and a pinch of cumin seeds. Pour over 65 grams of couscous, cover and leave to stand until it has absorbed the liquid. Remove the chicken from the marinade, spray with Fry Light and grill under high heat for 4 minutes each side. Serve with the couscous, plenty of steamed broccoli, and a fresh parsley garnish if you like.

300 calories   5 grams of fat

4. Oriental Salmon

Mix 2 tablespoons of teriyaki sauce with 125 ml orange juice. Place two 100-gram salmon steaks in a large frying pan, pour over the sauce, bring to the boil and then reduce the heat.

Cover and cook for 3–5 minutes until the salmon is cooked through. Remove the fish and keep warm. Mix a teaspoon of cornflour with a tablespoon of water until smooth, stir into the orange sauce and cook over a gentle heat until thickened. Meanwhile, quickly cook 200 grams of glass noodles. Pour the sauce over the salmon and serve with the glass noodles and a large portion of beansprouts (canned beansprouts are quick to heat on the hob or in the microwave).

350 calories   13 grams of fat

5. Fisherman's Stew
Bake 2 large baking potatoes in the oven. Half an hour before they are ready, chop an onion and a clove of garlic. Heat a large, non-stick pan, spray with a few shots of Fry Light and cook the onion and garlic for 3–4 minutes until soft. Meanwhile, chop 1 stick of celery and cut 1 large carrot into thin sticks. Add these to the softened onion and garlic along with a pinch of fennel seeds and a 400-gram can of chopped tomatoes. Bring to the boil and simmer for 5 minutes. Add 300 grams of fresh or frozen fillets of cod. Cook for 5 minutes if fresh and 10 if frozen. Add a handful of chopped fresh coriander and season with salt and pepper. Split open the potato and remove the flesh. Sprinkle the flesh with lemon juice and black pepper, then fluff up and return to the skins. Serve with the stew.

350 calories   7 grams of fat

6. Quick Micro-Mustard Chicken
Combine 1 tablespoon of Dijon mustard with 1 teaspoon of mixed dried herbs and 2 dessertspoons of plain yoghurt. Arrange two 150-gram skinless chicken breasts in a microwaveable dish – thickest parts towards the outside of the dish. Spread the yoghurt and mustard sauce over chicken and grind over some black pepper. Microwave on high for 4 minutes; if the chicken is still pink inside, microwave a little longer. Serve with 200 grams of boiled new potatoes, and baby corn and carrot chunks, or any two of your favourite vegetables.

300 calories   6 grams of fat

7. Seafood Spaghetti

Heat 1 dessertspoon of olive oil in a large pan and gently cook a medium-sized chopped onion for 4 minutes. Add a 400-gram can of chopped tomatoes, 1 crushed garlic clove, 1 bay leaf and a pinch each of dried basil and oregano. Stir in 1 small can (140 grams) of clams and a dash of Worcestershire sauce. Simmer for 5 minutes. Serve with the pasta of your choice (this sauce works well with spaghetti): 70 grams for each of you.

400 calories   7 grams of fat

8. Quick Macaroni Pie

Cook 140 grams of macaroni in a large pot of boiling, salted water. When cooked and drained, place in a large ovenproof dish. Add 1 chopped fresh red chilli, 1 finely chopped onion, the juice of 1 lemon, 2 tablespoons of tomato ketchup, 1 teaspoon of dried or fresh marjoram and 1 teaspoon of dried sage, and combine well with the cooked macaroni. Beat 1 egg with 100 ml skimmed milk and pour over the macaroni. Sprinkle 1 tablespoon of grated half-fat Cheddar over the top, and bake for 25–30 minutes in a preheated moderate oven (180°C/gas 4). Mix some salad leaves with 2 tablespoons of tinned drained sweetcorn and some sliced red or green pepper and use to garnish the macaroni pie.

350 calories   6 grams of fat

9. Stir-Fried Pork with Mangetout

Cut 200 grams of extra-lean pork into strips and put into a bowl with 2 teaspoons of Lea and Perrins ginger sauce (or a pinch of ground ginger), 1 chopped shallot, 1 teaspoon of finely crushed coriander seeds, 1 crushed garlic clove and 2 teaspoons of lemon juice. Leave covered for one hour. Put 120 grams of rice on to cook. Meanwhile, heat 1 teaspoon of oil in a wok or large frying pan. Add the pork and its marinade and stir-fry briskly for 3–5 minutes until cooked through. Add 50 grams of mangetout or sugarsnap peas and a carrot cut into strips. Cook for 2 minutes then pour in 150 ml of hot stock. Blend a teaspoon of cornflour with a little water and add to the pan. Heat until sauce thickens, then serve with the rice.

290 calories   8 grams of fat

10. *Sweet and Sour Pork*
Chop 1 onion, de-seed and dice 1/2 green pepper, slice 1 carrot, crush 1 clove of garlic and drain a 100-gram can of water chestnuts. Heat a non-stick frying pan or wok and spray with a shot of Fry Light. Add the onion, green pepper, carrot, garlic and water chestnuts and stir-fry for 3–4 minutes, then add a few tablespoons of water and keep cooking for another 4 minutes. Remove from the pan and set aside. Wipe briskly around the pan with kitchen paper. Spray two 100-gram extra lean pork fillets with a shot of Fry Light and cook in the pan for 3 minutes each side, spraying again as you turn. Meanwhile, dissolve 2 teaspoons of cornflour in 1 1/2 tablespoons of vinegar. Add 1 tablespoon of water, 1 teaspoon of soy sauce and 1 tablespoon of brown sugar. Drain into this the natural juice from a 100-gram can of pineapple chunks. Add this sauce mixture to the pork and cook for 2 minutes so that it thickens. Stir in the onion mix and the pineapple chunks and cook for another 2 minutes. Serve with a large baked potato topped with a tablespoon of low-fat fromage frais and black pepper.

350 calories   4 grams of fat

11. *Mild Chicken, Corn and Potato Curry*
Chop 1 onion and 1 clove of garlic. Heat a non-stick frying pan, spray with a shot of Fry Light and cook the onion and garlic for 3 minutes. Meanwhile, scrub and chop 160 grams of unpeeled potato, and chop 180 grams of chicken breast. Add 1 teaspoon of curry powder to the onion and garlic, stir well and cook briefly, then add the chopped chicken breast and potato. Stir in a handful of raisins and a teaspoon of freshly grated ginger (grated from frozen for ease) and remove from the heat. Transfer to a large ovenproof dish. Dissolve 1/2 teaspoon of cornflour with 1 teaspoon of lemon juice and pour into the chicken along with a 150-gram carton of low-fat yoghurt.

Slowly whisk in 150 ml of chicken stock (made with a cube). Cook in a moderate oven (180°C/gas 4) for 50 minutes. Serve with 2 poppadoms that have been microwaved for 60 seconds, and garnish the dish with chopped mixed peppers.

300 calories   5 grams of fat

12. Gnocchi with Olive Tomato Sauce

Buy ready-made gnocchi and weigh out 300 grams. Chop 1 onion and 1 clove of garlic. Heat a non-stick pan, spray with a shot of Fry Light and quickly cook through the onion and garlic. Add a 400-gram can of chopped tomatoes with basil, a dash of Worcestershire sauce and 4 stoned black olives and 4 green olives cut into quarters. Cook for 8 minutes, adding a pinch of salt, pepper and a teaspoon of sugar when nearly ready. Meanwhile, boil the gnocchi for 3–4 minutes. Drain, divide between 2 hot plates and top with the sauce. Grind over some black pepper and 2 teaspoons each of grated Parmesan. Serve with a green salad.

400 calories   4 grams of fat

13. Sausage and Horseradish Mash

Boil 300 grams of potatoes. While they are cooking, start to grill 3 Quorn sausages. Cut 2 tomatoes in half and sprinkle with Worcestershire sauce, and spray a couple of mushrooms with Fry Light. Add the tomatoes and mushrooms to the grill pan, and turn the sausages. Mash the boiled potatoes with semi-skimmed milk to taste, 2 teaspoons of horseradish sauce, 2 teaspoons of mustard and salt and black pepper. Serve the mashed potatoes with the sausages, mushrooms and tomatoes.

350 calories   6 grams of fat

14. Trout in a Foil Bag

Boil 300 grams of new potatoes with a sprig of mint. While they are cooking, season 2 trout fillets, 120 grams each, with salt and black pepper and brush with lemon juice. Cut 2 large ovals of tin foil and spray each on the inside with 2 shots of Fry Light. Place a little finely chopped spring onion, carrot and courgette on each foil then lay the trout over. Pour 2 tablespoons of white wine or stock over each fillet. Fold over the tin foil and crumple the edges so that each packet is airtight. Bake in a moderate oven (180°C/gas 4) for 8 minutes. Remove from the oven and the foil. Serve with the new potatoes.

300 calories   6 grams of fat

15. 'Sunday' Roast

Serve yourself 100 grams of roast chicken or lean roast pork, minus the skin or crackling. Cover with a gravy made from cornflour and stock and surround with a mound of vegetables including two small roast potatoes (75 grams in total), a roast parsnip and as many lightly steamed vegetables such as carrots, sprouts, broccoli, cauliflower or cabbage as you can manage.

390 calories   14 grams of fat

16. Ham, Egg and Chips

Cook 100 grams of oven chips. Cut two tomatoes in half and grill. When the chips are almost ready, spray a non-stick pan with Fry Light and fry a large egg. Serve the egg and chips with a 40-gram slice of lean ham and your favourite sauce: brown, ketchup – it's up to you.

400 calories   16 grams of fat

17. Shepherd's Pie

Boil 250 grams of peeled potatoes for mashing. In a non-stick frying pan brown 180 grams of extra lean minced lamb. Transfer to a bowl and blot off the fat with kitchen paper. In a saucepan combine a small, finely chopped onion, a clove of crushed garlic, 225 ml of stock, 1 tablespoon of tomato purée and a dash each of soy and Worcestershire sauce. Simmer for 10 minutes until the stock is reduced, then add the lamb. Season with salt, pepper and a pinch of nutmeg and add a further 150 ml of stock. Simmer for 15 minutes. Mash the potatoes with skimmed milk to taste and black pepper. Place the meat in a medium-sized casserole dish, spread over the mashed potato and flash under a hot grill until the potato lightly browns. Serve with freshly cooked spring greens and other vegetables if you like.

350 calories   15 grams of fat

18. Quick Pilaf

Heat a non-stick pan, spray with a shot of Fry Light and add 80 grams of extra lean cubed beef (or gammon if you prefer), a finely chopped onion and a crushed clove of garlic. Cook for about 5 minutes, stirring frequently. Meanwhile, finely dice 2 carrots and 2 sticks of celery. To the meat add 100 grams of long-grain rice, the diced carrot and celery, 2 teaspoons of sultanas, a pinch of allspice and a bay leaf. Pour over 250 ml of boiling chicken stock (made with a cube). Cover the pan and cook for 15 to 20 minutes. Stir in 4 tablespoons of frozen peas and 2 chopped tomatoes and cook for a further minute. Check the seasoning and consistency. If too sloppy, cook a little longer. Remove the bay leaf before serving.

350 calories   5 grams of fat

19. Grilled Sardines with Lemon

Buy 4 large, cleaned and gutted sardines. Once home, run them under water, then spray with Fry Light and sprinkle with lemon juice and black pepper. Cook under a hot grill for 3–4 minutes each side. Arrange on a warmed serving dish decorated with parsley along with wedges of lemon to squeeze over. Serve with a 50-gram chunk of hot crusty bread each and a tomato salad with balsamic vinegar.

400 calories   21 grams of fat

20. Trout with Caramelized Onions

Cook 300 grams of new potatoes in boiling salted water until tender. Slice 2 onions. Heat a non-stick frying pan and spray with a shot of Fry Light. Add the onions and 1 teaspoon of brown sugar, and cook for 5 minutes until the onions start to caramelize. Drain and slice the potatoes and, in a bowl, pour 50 ml of vegetable stock and 1 tablespoon of white wine vinegar over them while they're stll warm. Toss gently and sprinkle with plenty of chopped fresh parsley. Spray two 100-gram trout fillets with Fry Light and cook under a hot grill for 3 minutes each side. Serve the potato salad with the trout, caramelized onions and 6 stoned black olives.

300 calories   6 grams of fat

21. Aromatic Salmon

Season two 90-gram salmon fillets well with salt, black pepper and the grated zest of a lemon. Place the salmon in a bamboo steamer with a crushed stick of lemongrass and a crushed piece of ginger. Steam for 6 minutes. Heat a non-stick frying pan and spray with Fry Light. Add 180 grams of fresh beansprouts and sauté quickly with 1 teaspoon each of fish sauce and soy sauce. Cook 300 grams of fresh noodles. Serve the noodles and beansprouts immediately with the steamed salmon.

300 calories   13 grams of fat

22. Rosemary Turkey Grill

Into 50 ml of orange juice stir 1 teaspoon of dried rosemary, some freshly ground black pepper and 1 crushed garlic clove. Put two 150-gram turkey breasts in a shallow dish and pour over the flavoured juice. Cover and leave for 10 minutes in the kitchen or for 1 hour in the fridge, remembering to turn the turkey over halfway through. Heat the grill and remove the turkey from the marinade. Grill for 3–4 minutes either side, basting with the remaining marinade as it cooks. Serve with 300 grams of boiled new potatoes and puréed carrots.

300 calories   3 grams of fat

23. Poached Cod and Beansprouts

Heat 200 ml skimmed milk with a bay leaf, some thyme and a clove of garlic, then poach two 110-gram pieces of skinned cod slowly for 6 minutes. (If you use frozen fillets, cook as long as packet instructs.) Heat a non-stick frying pan, spray with 2 shots of Fry Light and sauté 100 grams of fresh beansprouts. After 3 minutes, add a few dashes of balsamic vinegar to the pan, then turn onto warmed serving plates. Remove the cod from its poaching liquid and place on top. Sprinkle with chopped fresh parsley and serve with warm chunks of bread (55 grams each) and lemon wedges to squeeze over.

300 calories   3 grams of fat

24. Quick Fish Bake with Mash

Place two 150-gram cod or haddock steaks in an ovenproof dish. Finely chop 1 leek and a handful of fresh parsley, and roughly chop 4 mushrooms. Heat a non-stick frying pan, spray with a shot of Fry Light and stir-fry the leek briefly. Add the mushrooms and parsley, and pour in 115ml of canned condensed mushroom soup. Stir until the soup starts to boil, then pour this over the fish steaks, cover and bake at 190°C/gas 5 for 30 minutes. Meanwhile, boil 200 grams of potatoes until tender. Drain and mash with skimmed milk to taste and seasoning. Just before the fish bake is ready, quickly cook 100 grams of frozen peas. Serve the bake with the peas and mash.

350 calories   8 grams of fat

25. Piri Piri Chicken Fillets

Take two 120-gram boned and skinned chicken fillets and cut through lengthways so that you can open each one out flat. Mix together in a bowl 1 finely sliced stick of celery, some crushed garlic, a pinch of piri piri or chilli powder and some salt and pepper. Divide the mix in two and use to stuff the chicken fillets. Secure with a cocktail stick. Mix 1 tablespoon of balsamic vinegar with 1 tablespoon of honey, 1 teaspoon of olive oil, a good pinch of dried dill and some salt and pepper. Brush some of this over the chicken and then cook under a hot grill for 15–20 minutes, turning 3 or 4 times and brushing with the remaining balsamic vinegar mix. Serve with 250 grams of new boiled potatoes and 150 grams of mangetout or sugarsnap peas.

300 calories   8 grams of fat

26. *Tangy Cheese Patties*
Boil 400 grams of potatoes until tender and steam 200 grams of shredded cabbage until likewise. Drain the potatoes and mash with the cabbage, a few chopped spring onions and 50 grams of grated halt-fat mature Cheddar. Divide the mix into quarters and shape into cakes. Preheat the grill and spray the patties with Fry Light. Grill for 5 minutes, turn, spray again and grill for a further 2 minutes. Make a tangy chutney by mixing together 3 tablespoons of apricot jam with a few drops of chilli sauce and 2 teaspoons of cider vinegar. Serve the patties with the chutney and a large green salad with fat-free vinaigrette.

300 calories   5 grams of fat

27. *Speedy Beany Casserole*
Boil 200 grams of potatoes until tender, then drain and set aside. Meanwhile, chop an onion and dice a stick of celery. Heat 1 teaspoon of oil in a frying pan and cook the onion and celery for a few minutes, stirring to prevent sticking. Add 200 grams of canned, drained red kidney beans, 200 grams of canned, drained brown lentils and 200 grams of canned tomatoes with garlic and herbs. Stir in a dash of Lea and Perrins garlic and chilli sauce or Worcestershire sauce. Heat thoroughly until it simmers. Slice the potatoes and place in the bottom of two individual bowls, then pour over the bean mix. Top each with 1 tablespoon of grated reduced-fat Cheddar and serve.

380 calories   7 grams of fat

28. *Chicken Satay with Pittas*
Mix 1 teaspoon of peanut butter with 3 tablespoons of lemon juice, 1 tablespoon of soy sauce, 1 tablespoon of water, 1 teaspoon of honey, a pinch of chilli powder and a crushed garlic clove. Put two 100-gram skinless chicken breasts into a shallow dish and pour over the mix. Leave for 10 minutes. Grate the zest of an orange and mix with its juice. Grate 2 carrots and stir into the orange juice along with 1 teaspoon of mustard and 1 teaspoon of poppy seeds. Remove the chicken

from the marinade and place on a grill pan. Brush with the marinade and cook under a hot grill for 4 minutes each side. Warm two mini pittas under the grill and serve the chicken and pittas with the orange carrot salad.

300 calories   6 grams of fat

Five-minute Lunches

Egg Mayo Sarnie
Mix a chopped, cold, hardboiled egg with 1 tablespoon of reduced-calorie salad cream and lots of freshly ground black pepper. Make into a sandwich with 2 slices of wholemeal bread. Add shredded lettuce and or mustard and cress.

300 calories   11 grams of fat

Cheddar Pickle Roll
Spread a roll with pickle. Fill with 35 grams of grated reduced-fat mature Cheddar mixed with a finely chopped spring onion and topped with slices of cucumber.

300 calories   9 grams of fat

Mustard Mackerel Toasts
Mash a can of mackerel fillets in mustard sauce with some chopped onion. Spread over two thick slices of toast and serve with a large green salad.

350 calories   14 grams of fat

Potato Waffles
Grill 2 potato waffles for 6 minutes, turning once. Top with 50 grams of canned sardines in tomato sauce mashed with some vinegar (balsamic if you have it); 40 grams of grated reduced-fat Cheddar; and 115ml baked beans or 100 grams of your favourite flavoured cottage cheese. Serve with a large mixed green salad. All these versions are low in fat and supply around 300 calories.

Camembert Ploughman's
Arrange all the following on a plate and serve: 50-gram chunk of Camembert cheese, 1 tablespoon of pickle, 3 pickled onions, 1 tomato cut into sections, and some chunks of cucumber and lettuce leaves.

300 calories   14 grams of fat

Meat Sandwiches
Spread two slices of bread with reduced-fat salad cream. Fill with 70 to 80 grams of cooked chicken, turkey, lean pork or lean beef. Add plenty of salad to bulk out the sandwich plus ground black pepper for flavour. All these options are low in fat and supply around 300 calories.

Easy Baked Spuds
Bake a 150-gram baking potato in the oven or microwave. Split open the potato and spoon out the soft flesh. Mix the potato flesh with lemon juice and black pepper, then fluff up and return to the skin. Add any of the following:

  small can of baked beans
   100 grams of cottage cheese of your choice
   40 grams of chopped ham mixed with 50 grams of very low-fat fromage frais and a tomato
   60 grams of prawns mixed with 1 tablespoon of Thousand Island dressing and 2 tablespoons of low-fat yoghurt
   40 grams of grated reduced-fat Cheddar
   and serve with a large green salad with fat-free vinaigrette dressing. All these options are low in fat and supply around 300 calories.

Take-away Sandwiches
Any 300-calorie ready-made sandwich from Boots, Tesco, Asda, Safeway, Sainsbury's, Marks & Spencer or Somerfield.

Quick Dinners

Micro Meals
Buy any of the 300-calorie ready-made dinners, either chilled or frozen, and serve with lightly steamed or boiled vegetables of your

choice, such as carrots, broccoli, cauliflower, greens or sprouts. Alternatively, serve with a green salad with fat-free dressing.

Fast Chicken Korma

Cut 100 grams of skinless chicken breast into chunks. Heat a non-stick pan, spray with a shot of Fry Light and brown the chicken, stirring frequently. Mix 100 grams of Uncle Ben's Light Chicken Korma into half an individual pot of plain yoghurt and add to the chicken. Cover and simmer for 30 minutes. Add a little chicken stock if necessary. Serve with a third of a can of Uncle Ben's canned Express rice (about 90 grams) or a similar amount of standard rice.

350 calories   10 grams of fat

Pork Stir-Fry

Cut 100 grams of lean pork into strips. Heat a non-stick frying pan or wok, spray with a few shots of Fry Light and add the pork. Stir-fry for 3 minutes, adding a dash of soy sauce and a little grated ginger and crushed garlic if you have some. After 3 minutes add as much frozen vegetable stir-fry mix as you think you can manage. Stir-fry for a further 4 minutes, adding some more soy sauce and a little stock if necessary to moisten. Serve with half a can of Uncle Ben's Express canned rice (about 140 grams).

400 calories   5 grams of fat

Ten-Minute Pasta

Cook 75 grams of pasta and serve with a low-fat tomato pasta sauce such as Paul Newman's Sockarooni or Dolmio Light. Serve with a green salad and fat-free dressing.

300 calories   3 grams of fat

Chicken Chop Suey

Finely slice 100 grams of lean, skinned chicken breast. Heat a non-stick frying pan, spray with a shot of Fry Light and brown the chicken. Remove the chicken, spray again, and add some chopped mushrooms, beansprouts and a dash of soy sauce. Stir-fry for about 1 minute then add half a jar of Sharwoods Chop

Suey Stir-Fry sauce. Heat through and serve with a 100-gram pack of Batchelors Super Noodles, which you make just by pouring on boiling water.

400 calories   13 grams of fat

Cauliflower Cheese
Serves 1

Cook a small cauliflower. Make up a white sauce using a packet of mix and 250 ml skimmed milk. Stir in a teaspoon of English mustard and 20 grams of grated reduced-fat mature Cheddar. Pour the sauce over the cauliflower, sprinkle with 20 grams of reduced-fat Cheddar and brown under the grill. Serve with a 50-gram chunk of bread or a roll.

400 calories   11 grams of fat

100-Calorie Snacks
Bread and so on:
   1 toasted crumpet with jam
   1 slice of medium-sized toast with jam
   1 slice of malt bread
   1 Scotch pancake with jam

Biscuits and cakes:
   1 Go Ahead double chocolate cake bar (McVitie's)
   2 Jaffa cakes
   1 fig roll
   1 digestive
   2 ginger nuts
   5 sponge fingers
   1 Boots forest fruit cereal bar
   1 slice of Swiss roll or 1 mini Swiss roll
   1 98 per cent fat-free chocolate brownie (California Cake and Cookie Company)
   1 98 per cent fat-free carrot cake (California Cake and Cookie Company)
   1 piece Madeira cake

Sweets:
   1 Boots Shapers Turkish delight bar
   1 Boots Shapers cappuccino, caramel, coconut, crispy
      caramel or mint bar
   60 grams of fruit gums
   40 grams of fruit pastilles
   25 grams of mints
   1 Ferrero Rocher
   1 fun-size Maltesers, Milky Way, M&Ms or Mars
   1 Halo bar
   1 standard Milky Bar
   3 After Eights
   2 Black Magic
   5 Match Makers
   2 Quality Street sweets

Puddings:
   1 Boots Shapers raspberry trifle
   1 M&S Strawberry Fool Lite
   1 individual carton of Ambrosia banana-flavour dessert
   100 grams of rice pudding made with skimmed milk
   1 Shapers banana split sundae
   50-gram Arctic roll
   140 grams of Too Good To Be True ice cream
   1 strawberry split ice lolly
   1 dark choc ice (40 grams) from Tesco
   1 Opal Fruits ice lolly
   55 grams of scoop ice cream
   75 grams of scoop sorbet
   90 grams of Orchard Maid raspberry or strawberry luxury
      frozen yoghurt
   90 grams of crème caramel
   150 grams of jelly
   1 Asda Farm Stores 125-gram low-fat yoghurt
   1 Boots Shapers split yoghurts
   200-gram Co-op light yoghurt
   1 Eden Vale French-style yoghurt
   125-gram Loseley very-low fat yoghurt

200-gram pot Müller Light
1 Ski extra-fruit low-fat yoghurt

Crisps and savoury snacks:
1 packet Boots Shapers prawn shells
1 packet Boots Shapers American barbecue waffles
20 Snyder's mini fat-free pretzels
1 toasted crumpet with Marmite
1 Sainsbury's potato cake (toasted) with Marmite
1/2 pack of Tesco's fresh chunky tomato soup
1/2 pack of Asda's fresh tomato and basil soup
1/3 pack 95 per cent fat-free potato salad
100 grams of Sainsbury's 95 per cent fat-free mint and lemon couscous salad
50 grams of Shape cherry, tomato and basil cottage cheese with 3 Harvest Slim crispbreads

50-Calorie Snacks
Fruits:
150 grams of apricots
50 grams of banana (1/2 average banana)
200 grams of blackberries
100 grams of cherries
130 grams of damsons
35 grams of dates
1 fresh fig
150 grams of grapefruit
90 grams of grapes
200 grams of guava
100 grams of lychees
100 grams of mango
200 grams of cantaloupe melon
200 grams of honeydew melon
200 grams of watermelon
130 grams of mulberries
1 nectarine
130 grams of oranges
130 grams of pawpaw (papaya)

140 grams of peach
120 grams of pear
140 grams of plums
200 grams of raspberries
100 grams of rhubarb stewed with sugar
200 grams of strawberries

Others:
1 Danone Petite fromage frais
1 Holland & Barrett Diet Yoghurt
100-gram pot of Safeway virtually fat-free fromage frais
100-gram pot of St Ivel Lite fromage frais
100g Shape fromage frais
100-gram pot of Weight Watchers from Heinz fromage frais
40-gram tube of Yoplait Frubes
1 Cadbury's Mini Caramel Egg, Mini Cream Egg
1 Aero mini bar
1 mini Bounty
2 Buttermints, barley sugars, boiled fruit sweets

Alcohol
275ml bottle of lager
275ml bottle of stout
275ml bottle of pale ale
1/2 pint dry cider
1 glass wine (115ml)
2 × 1/3 gill dry or medium sherry
1/6 gill liqueurs, brandy or whisky

ENJOY IT, KEEP IT UP, AND GOOD LUCK